IMAGING
IN STROKE

Editor:
Michael G. Hennerici

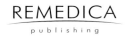
REMEDICA
publishing

LONDON • CHICAGO

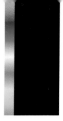

Contributors

Editor

Michael G. Hennerici, MD
Professor
Department of Neurology
University of Heidelberg
Universitätsklinikum Mannheim
Theodor-Kutzer-Ufer
D-68135 Mannheim
Germany

Authors

Julien Bogousslavsky, MD
Professor
Department of Neurology
Centre Hospitalier Universitaire
Vaudois
Lausanne
Switzerland

Gabriel R. de Freitas, MD
Department of Neurology
Universidade Federal do Rio de Janeiro
Rio de Janeiro
Brazil

Wolf-Dieter Heiss, MD
Professor
Department of Neurology, University of
Cologne, and Max-Planck Institute for
Neurological Research
Gleuelerstr. 50
D-50931 Cologne
Germany

Michael G. Hennerici, MD
Professor
Department of Neurology
University of Heidelberg
Universitätsklinikum Mannheim
Theodor-Kutzer-Ufer
D-68135 Mannheim
Germany

Olav Jansen, MD
Professor
Section of Neuroradiology
Department of Neurosurgery
University of Kiel
Weimarerstr. 8
D-24106 Kiel
Germany

Christoph Koch, MD
Department of Neuroradiology
University Hospital Schleswig-Holstein
Ratzeburger Allee 160
D-23538 Lübeck
Germany

Thomas Kucinski, MD
Department of Neuroradiology
University-Hospital
Martinistr. 52
D-20246 Hamburg
Germany

Joachim Liepert, MD
Professor
Department of Neurology
University Hospital Eppendorf
Martinistr. 52
D-20246 Hamburg
Germany

Stephen Meairs, Priv-Doz, MD
Department of Neurology
Universitätsklinikum Mannheim
D-68135 Mannheim
Germany

Michael Moseley, PhD
Professor of Radiology
Department of Radiology
Stanford University
1201 Welch Road
Lucas Center, P286
Stanford, California 94305-5488
USA

Tobias Neumann-Haefelin, MD
Klinik für Neurologie
Johann Wolfgang von Goethe –
Universität
Schleusenweg 2-16
D-60528 Frankfurt
Germany

Fabienne Perren, MD
Department of Neurology
CHUV
Lausanne
Switzerland

Cornelius Weiller, MD
Professor
Head of the Department of Neurology
University Hospital Eppendorf
Martinistr. 52
D-20246 Hamburg
Germany

Hermann Zeumer, MD
Professor
Chairman and Director of the
Department of Neuroradiology
University-Hospital
Martinistr. 52
D-20246 Hamburg
Germany

Contents

Preface

Our knowledge and experience with diagnostic imaging techniques is rapidly growing and has become increasingly important not only in the chronic but also in the acute stages of stroke. Following the approval of specific treatment strategies for ischemic stroke – and with strong evidence indicating the likelihood of a similar development for hemorrhagic stroke – diagnostic accuracy is becoming increasingly essential in order to tailor management for the individual patient. Neurologists and stroke physicians need to familiarize themselves with the prolific advances that imaging has made to our understanding of the pathophysiology of stroke and the ability of available technologies to image brain and vascular tissue changes at onset and during stroke development. Application of this knowledge, particularly the relationship between imaging data and clinical signs and symptoms – and the patient's history – coupled with an awareness of the limitations of imaging, is essential for optimal, rapid and safe management of stroke patients.

Progress with neuroimaging techniques in the visualization of cerebrovascular changes (ultrasound, computed tomography-angiography, and magnetic resonance angiography) and in the understanding of brain tissue metabolism (magnetic resonance imaging and positron emission tomography) has redefined the nature of stroke as a dynamic and evolving process. This knowledge has ignited the quest for greater diagnostic accuracy and – in line with evidence-based interpretation of clinical study results – suggests that the technical management of stroke patients should be regularly remodelled to take into account updated evidence-based data from imaging studies.

This book is designed to provide practical and ready access to these diagnostic approaches to stroke syndromes, with particular emphasis on technical studies and their correlation with clinical findings – in both acute and chronic stages of the disease. In this time of rapid methodological development, we hope that this book will equip physicians with a better understanding of the different imaging techniques and their interrelated advantages and pitfalls.

Michael G. Hennerici
Mannheim, Spring 2003

1

Classification of stroke

Gabriel R. de Freitas & Julien Bogousslavsky

Historical aspects

From the time of Hippocrates, cerebral infarction, intracerebral hemorrhage, and subarachnoid hemorrhage were all termed 'apoplexy', the old word for stroke. It was only in 1658, when Wepfer demonstrated that apoplexy was caused by hemorrhage, and, almost two centuries later, in 1823, when Rostan linked 'softening of the brain' to disease of the arteries, that the two major mechanisms of stroke, 'plugs and leaks', were identified [1]. The initial recognition of the mechanisms of cerebral infarction is credited to Virchow (1856), Gowers (1885), Chiari (1905), and Ramsay Hunt (1914), who put forward the concepts of atherosclerosis of the cervical vessels and embolism [1]. However, these received little attention in the first half of the 20th century until reappraised by Miller Fisher, who, in a landmark paper, gave a detailed description of eight patients with infarcts due to carotid obstruction [2]. It was also Miller Fisher who was responsible, between 1965 and the 1990s, for refinements of the concepts of lacunae [3,4], small infarcts in the deep white matter first studied by French investigators in the 1830s [5].

One of the earliest attempts to classify cerebrovascular disease using *in vivo* characteristics is attributed to Millikan et al. [6], who divided the disease into three major categories: cerebral infarction, transient focal cerebral ischemic attacks without infarction, and intracranial hemorrhage. Cerebral infarction was further subdivided into thrombosis with stenosis, cerebral embolism, other conditions causing cerebral infarction, and cerebral infarction of undetermined type. Further epidemiological studies and stroke registries divided intracranial hemorrhage into intracerebral hemorrhage and subarachnoid hemorrhage [7,8]. The classification used in the Harvard Cooperative Stroke Registry, published in 1978, incorporated lacunae as a subtype of cerebral infarction [8]. The classifications of the Lausanne Stroke Registry (LSR) [9] and the Oxford Community Stroke Project (OCSP) [10] provided a better delineation of the

Cerebral infarction subtype	Criteria
Atherosclerosis with stenosis	Narrowing ≥ 50% of the lumen diameter of the corresponding extracranial artery or large intracranial artery (MCA, PCA, or basilar artery), in the absence of another etiology
Atherosclerosis without stenosis	Plaques or <50% stenosis of the corresponding extracranial artery or large intracranial artery, in the absence of another etiology and in patients with at least two of the following five risk factors: age ≥ 50 years, hypertension, diabetes mellitus, cigarette smoking, or hypercholesterolemia
Emboligenic heart disease	Intracardiac thrombus or tumor, rheumatic mitral stenosis, prosthetic aortic or mitral valve, endocarditis, atrial fibrillation, sick sinus syndrome, left ventricular aneurysm or akinesia after myocardial infarction, acute (<3 months) myocardial infarction, or global cardiac hypokinesia or dyskinesia, in the absence of another etiology
Hypertensive arteriolopathy	Infarction in the territory of a deep perforating artery in a patient with known hypertension, in the absence of another etiology
Mixed etiologies	Combination of the above four etiologies
Other etiologies	Arterial dissection, fibromuscular dysplasia, saccular aneurysm, AVM, cerebral venous thrombosis on angiography, angiitis (multiple segmental arterial narrowing on angiography, pleocytosis of the CSF), hematologic conditions (polycythemia, thrombocythemia, etc.), migraine (history of migraine, occurrence of stroke during an attack of migraine), or other
Undetermined	None of the above causes of cerebral infarction could be determined

AVM: arteriovenous malformation; CSF: cerebrospinal fluid; MCA: middle carotid artery; PCA: posterior carotid artery.

Table 1. The Lausanne Stroke Registry classification.

criteria for infarct subtypes, including a more precise definition of the subgroups of large-artery disease and lacunar infarction (**Tables 1** and **2**). Most stroke classifications used today, such as the Trial of Org 10172 in Acute Stroke Treatment (TOAST) classification (**Table 3**) [11], use the core mechanistic grouping present in the earlier classifications [12]. In this chapter, we will focus on the methods and shortcomings of the classifications of cerebral infarction.

Infarction subtype	Criteria
LACI	Pure motor stroke (i.e., weakness of face and limbs on one side of the body without abnormalities of higher brain function, sensation, or vision); pure sensory stroke (i.e., decreased sensation of face and limbs on one side of the body without abnormalities of higher brain function, sensation, or vision); sensorimotor stroke (i.e., weakness and decreased sensation of face and limbs on one side of the body without abnormalities of higher brain function, sensation, or vision); or ataxic hemiparesis (i.e., weakness and ataxia of face and limbs on one side of the body without abnormalities of higher brain function, sensation, or vision)
TACI	Combination of new higher cerebral dysfunction (e.g., aphasia, dyscalculia, visuospatial disorder); homonymous visual field defect; and ipsilateral motor and/or sensory deficit of at least two areas of the face, arm, and leg. If the conscious level was impaired and formal testing of higher cerebral function or the visual fields was not possible, a deficit was assumed
PACI	Two of the three components of the TACI syndrome, with higher cerebral dysfunction alone, or with a motor/sensory deficit more restricted than those classified as LACI (e.g., confined to one limb, or to face and hand but not to the whole arm)
POCI	Any of the following: ipsilateral cranial nerve palsy with contralateral motor and/or sensory deficit; bilateral motor and/or sensory deficit; disorder of conjugate eye movement; cerebellar dysfunction without ipsilateral long-tract deficit (i.e., ataxic hemiparesis); or isolated homonymous visual field defect

LACI: lacunar infarcts; PACI: partial anterior circulation infarcts; POCI: posterior circulation infarcts; TACI: total anterior circulation infarcts.

Table 2. The Oxfordshire Community Stroke Project classification.

Main classifications

The classification of stroke into categories and subcategories is of great importance. The incidence of morbidity, mortality, and recurrence of hemorrhage and infarction in the various categories/subcategories is entirely different [13], as are their pathophysiology and natural history [14,15]. Therefore, an adequate classification is crucial not only for interchangeable use by investigators in different centers, but also for prevention, acute treatment, and definition of prognosis.

Cerebral infarction subtype	Criteria
Large-artery atherosclerosis	Clinical and brain imaging findings of either significant (>50%) stenosis or occlusion of a major brain artery or branch cortical artery, presumably due to atherosclerosis. Supportive evidence by duplex imaging or arteriography of a stenosis >50% of an appropriate intracranial or extracranial artery is needed. Diagnostic studies should exclude potential sources of cardiogenic embolism
Cardioembolism	Arterial occlusions presumably due to an embolus arising in the heart. Cardiac sources are divided into high-risk and medium-risk groups based on the evidence of their relative propensity for embolism

• High risk: mechanical prosthetic heart valve, mitral stenosis, atrial fibrillation (other than lone atrial fibrillation), left atrial/atrial appendage thrombus, sick sinus syndrome, recent (<4 weeks) myocardial infarction, left ventricular thrombus, dilated cardiomyopathy, akinetic left ventricular segment, atrial myxoma, infective endocarditis

• Medium risk: mitral valve prolapse, mitral annulus calcification, mitral stenosis without atrial fibrillation, left atrial turbulence (smoke), atrial septal aneurysm, patent foramen ovale, atrial flutter, lone atrial fibrillation, bioprosthetic heart valve, nonbacterial thrombotic endocarditis, congestive heart failure, hypokinetic left ventricular segment, myocardial infarction (>4 weeks, <6 months)

Potential large-artery atherosclerotic sources of thrombosis or embolism should be eliminated. A stroke in a patient with a medium-risk cardiac source of embolism and no other cause of stroke is classified as possible cardioembolic stroke |
Small-artery occlusion	The patient should have one of the traditional lacunar syndromes and should have no evidence of cerebral cortical dysfunction. The patient should also have a normal CT/MRI examination or a relevant brain stem or hemispheric lesion with a diameter <1.5 cm. Potential cardiac sources for emboli should be absent, and evaluation of the large extracranial arteries should not demonstrate a stenosis >50% in an ipsilateral artery
Other determined etiology	Patients with rare stroke causes, such as nonatherosclerotic vasculopathies, hypercoagulable states, or hematologic disorders
Stroke of undetermined etiology	Patients with no likely etiology despite an extensive evaluation (negative evaluation); patients with incomplete evaluation; and patients with two or more potential causes for the stroke

CT: computed tomography; MRI: magnetic resonance imaging.

Table 3. The Trial of Org 10172 in Acute Stroke Treatment (TOAST) classification.

Although some trials have reported efficacy of intervention regardless of the subtype of cerebral infarction [16,17], it seems logical that specific interventions (e.g., endarterectomy and intra-arterial thrombolysis) would only benefit patients with certain subtypes of infarcts [18,19]. Whether it is feasible to obtain a reliable classification during the acute stroke phase, within the current 3–6 hour therapeutic window, without increased expense and the limiting of therapy to specialized centers is still a matter of dispute [20,21].

The ideal classification should be simple, rapid enough to be applied in the acute stroke phase, capable of being applied to every patient, and based on the pathophysiologic mechanism of stroke. Moreover, it should provide good reliability, i.e., reproducibility of a measurement at two different points in time (intraobserver reliability) and between two or more observers (interobserver reliability).

All stroke classifications are artificial, relying on setting arbitrary limits for one or several characteristics of the stroke in order to allocate it to a specific category. Criteria used to differentiate subtypes of cerebral infarction include both clinical features that forecast the size and site of the lesion on computed tomography (CT) (e.g., the OCSP classification) and the probable etiology of stroke, based on risk factors and clinical features alone or combined with additional diagnostic studies, such as CT, magnetic resonance imaging (MRI), and Doppler ultrasonography (e.g., the LSR and TOAST classifications).

Unfortunately, distinguishing between cerebral infarction and hemorrhagic stroke, and between subtypes of cerebral infarction solely on clinical grounds is not easy. Neuroimaging (CT scan and novel MRI sequences) is the most accurate method of distinguishing cerebral hemorrhage from ischemia. However, at a time when few CT scanners were available and the technique was too expensive to be performed on every stroke patient, several scores (e.g., the Guy's Hospital and Siriraj scores) were developed to differentiate between these entities using clinical features alone [22–25]. But, when the validity of these scores was tested in populations in whom the frequency of hemorrhage was different from that observed in the original studies, they led to conflicting results, their predictive accuracy ranging from fair (64%) [26] to very good (93%) [27]. Although these scores seem to be useful in epidemiological studies, their utility in the clinical management of individual patients is disputable since therapeutic decisions should be made using methods with 100% accuracy, especially when considering more risky options such as thrombolysis and surgery.

LSR

The original classification, published in 1988, divides cerebral infarction into seven categories: atherosclerosis with stenosis (large-artery disease), atherosclerosis without stenosis, emb#oligenic heart disease, hypertensive arteriolopathy (small-vessel disease), mixed etiology, other etiology, and undetermined etiology (**Table 1**) [9]. In addition to the clinical findings, the systematic investigations carried out on all patients consist of brain imaging (CT and/or MRI), Doppler ultrasonography, electroencephalography (EEG), and standard blood and urine tests; while echocardiography, cerebral angiography, MR angiography, Holter, transcranial Doppler ultrasonography (TCD), and other examinations are performed on selected patients.

OCSP

Published in 1991, this classification divides cerebral infarction into four subgroups according to the presenting symptoms and signs: lacunar infarcts, total anterior circulation infarcts, partial anterior circulation infarcts, and posterior circulation infarcts (**Table 2**) [10]. Although this classification is not pathophysiologically based, it is simple, quick and, therefore, can be used in acute stroke. Other classifications based on size and site are related to specific mechanisms, and the authors stressed that classifications based on stroke mechanisms are time-consuming, impeding their use in the acute stroke phase, cannot be applied to those outpatients who do not undergo detailed investigation, and leave many patients with an undefined cause of stroke. However, in the acute stroke phase, only a moderate agreement (kappa = 0.41) between observers was obtained using the OCSP classification [28]. Differences in the assessment of some common neurologic signs result in only moderate (kappa = 0.39 for hemianopia) or poor (kappa = 0.15 for sensory loss) interobserver agreement [28].

TOAST

Published in 1993, this classification includes five categories: large-artery atherosclerosis, cardioembolism, small artery occlusion (lacune), stroke of other determined etiology, and stroke of undetermined etiology (**Table 3**) [12]. The diagnoses are based on clinical features and laboratory evaluations, such as brain imaging (CT or MRI), echocardiography, Doppler ultrasonography of extracranial arteries, arteriography, and an assessment of prothrombotic state. The authors argue that, in the acute phase, the physician can use the clinical and imaging findings to classify the stroke, and then reconsider this classification at a later stage when the results of other diagnostic tests are available. However, classification of stroke in the acute phase is quite difficult, and the initial clinical impression of stroke experts agreed with the final diagnosis in only 62% of cases in the TOAST study [29].

Main cerebral infarction subtypes

Cardioembolism
Epidemiology
Emboligenic heart disease was responsible for at least 20.4% (not including coexisting etiologies) of cerebral infarction cases in the LSR [9], and similar numbers were found in a population-based study [15]. Interestingly, the incidence of embolism is far higher in recent stroke registries or population-based studies than in those from a few decades ago [8,30]. Although one reason for this increase may be that, previously, strict clinical criteria had to be met for the diagnosis of cardioembolic stroke (i.e., rapidity of onset, previously recognized source, and coexistent systemic embolism [31]), the main reason is the development of new diagnostic tools, such as transthoracic and transesophageal echocardiography.

Etiology
The most common cardiac source of embolism in the LSR was abnormality of cardiac rhythm (49.1%, of which 92% were atrial fibrillation), followed by abnormality of the left ventricle wall (31.4%) or the aortic and mitral valves (26.9%) [32]. About one-fifth of patients had coexistent stroke causes (10.8% large-artery disease and 12.5% small-vessel disease).

Clinical findings
The clinical features associated with cardioembolism are an abrupt nonprogressive onset, isolated hemianopia, Wernicke's aphasia, and ideomotor apraxia [32]. In the National Institute of Neurological Disorders and Stroke (NINDS) Data Bank, cortical deficits (hemianopia, aphasia, and neglect) and a diminished level of consciousness were associated with cardiogenic embolism [33]. The carotid system territory was involved in 70% of patients, the vertebrobasilar area in 22%, a watershed area in 3%, and multiple infarcts in 5% [32]. In the Michael Reese Stroke Study, emboli lodged more frequently in the left middle cerebral artery (MCA) than in the right [30]. In the LSR, the anterior (19.7%) and posterior (17.7%) divisions of the MCA were equally involved, while, in patients with other stroke causes (e.g., large-artery disease), the posterior division was much less frequently involved than the anterior division [32]. Cardioembolism seems to be associated with more severe neurologic deficits at the time of the stroke and a poorer functional outcome compared to other stroke subtypes. In one study, mortality 1 month after stroke was four-times greater after cardioembolic stroke than after stroke due to large-artery disease [15].

Laboratory investigations
Thrombi were present on echocardiography in only 4% of patients with cardioembolism in the LSR [32], but the routine use of transthoracic

echocardiography might yield higher results. When performed in the acute stroke phase, angiography or TCD can document occlusion of the main trunk of the MCA or its major branches in the majority of patients [34]. Complete lysis of the occlusion occurs within hours to days, and is strongly suggestive of a cardioembolic, rather than an *in situ* thrombotic, mechanism [8,32,33].

Large-artery disease
Epidemiology
In the LSR, 24% of patients had a stroke due to large-artery (internal carotid artery [ICA] or large intracranial artery) stenosis or occlusion when strict criteria were used (>50% stenosis in the corresponding artery) [9]. When patients with large-artery stenosis, but without significant stenosis, and patients with coexisting stroke causes are also included, this figure increases to 43.2% of all infarcts. Atherosclerosis was probably an overestimated cause of infarctions in the past, when more than 70% of infarcts were attributed to it [35]. Stroke due to *in situ* atherosclerosis of the intracranial arteries is considered rare, but it may be of great importance in black or Japanese/Chinese patients [36].

Etiology
Large-artery disease may cause cerebral infarction by one of two different mechanisms: artery-to-artery emboli or hypoperfusion. The first is far more common, and, although the frequency of infarcts due to hypertension increases with increasing degree of ICA stenosis [37], embolism is still an important cause of stroke, even in internal carotid occlusion. In the setting of carotid occlusion, infarcts may be attributed to emboli from either an ulcerated stump or an ulcerated stenosis in the main collateral channels [38].

The pathogenesis of watershed infarcts is under debate [39–44]. The clinical evidence suggests that most of these are hemodynamic in nature, since events are commonly precipitated by an iatrogenic drop in blood pressure or standing up, loss of consciousness is observed at stroke onset, half of the patients have an elevated hematocrit, heart disease associated with hypotension is common (especially bradyarrhythmia), and most patients have occlusions or severe obstructions of the ipsilateral [40] and contralateral ICA [41]. However, embolism may be responsible in some cases and, in many instances, both embolism and hypoperfusion may play a role. It has been proposed that reduced blood flow at sites of arterial narrowing promotes the formation of thrombi and thus increases the risk of arterial thromboemboli. Another attractive hypothesis is that decreased perfusion reduces the washout and clearance of emboli that have entered the vascular bed of hypoperfused regions [42].

Clinical findings

The main territory involved in artery-to-artery emboli is the MCA: large-artery disease is responsible for 38% of complete MCA infarcts and 35% of MCA pial territory infarcts [9]. In addition, it is a substantial cause of cerebellar (29%) and brainstem (19%) infarcts. It should be stressed that in the LSR, it was associated with 16% of small deep infarcts (lacunae), thus arguing against the isolated role of lipohyalinosis in these infarcts. The most common clinical features are those of cortical involvement, but, in some instances, these can be misleading, e.g., in patients with classical lacunar syndromes, such as hemisensory impairment due to anterior parietal artery involvement (pseudothalamic syndrome of Foix) [44]. In a population-based study, these infarcts were associated with a higher rate of recurrence, especially in the acute phase [15].

Most watershed infarcts are in the anterior circulation, although they may also be present in the cerebellum, brainstem, and thalamus. The regions most often involved are the border zones between the middle and anterior cerebral arteries (anterior watershed infarcts), between the middle and posterior cerebral arteries (posterior watershed infarcts), and between the superficial and deep territories of the MCA (subcortical watershed infarcts).

Anterior watershed infarcts typically cause mainly crural hemiparesis, associated, in 50% of cases, with 'noncortical' hypoesthesia (elementary modes of sensation) in the same topography. Left-sided lesions are usually associated with transcortical motor aphasia, preceded by mutism, and right-sided lesions with mood disturbances (apathy or euphoria). Posterior watershed infarcts often cause macular sparing, incongruent hemianopia, and 'cortical' hypoesthesia (two-point discrimination, topoesthesia, and stereognosia), without hemiparesis. Anomia or transcortical sensory aphasia may be seen after left-sided lesions, while spatial neglect and anosognosia may be observed after right-sided infarcts. Subcortical watershed infarcts lead to hemiparesis, noncortical hemisensory defects, and language disorders in left-sided infarcts [40]. After severe hypotension (e.g., during cardiac surgery), bilateral lesions may be observed; when these involve the parieto-occipital region, Balint's syndrome (psychic gaze paralysis, optic ataxia, and visual inattention) may be observed [43].

Small-vessel disease

Epidemiology and etiology

This category accounted for 15% of the infarcts in the LSR [9], and a comparable percentage was observed in a subsequent study of a different population [15]. Pathological studies carried out in the 1960s by Fisher [4] emphasized that the lacunae were caused by 'segmental arterial disorganization', also called lipohyalinosis, a consequence of long-term hypertension.

Clinical findings

Small vessel disease can be divided into five classical lacunar syndromes (pure motor hemiparesis, pure sensory syndrome, sensorimotor stroke, ataxic hemiparesis, and ataxia-clumsy hand syndrome) [45,46]; although more than 70 distinct syndromes have been reported after lacunar lesions [47].

Patients with lacunar infarction often have a good prognosis. The fatality rate of lacunar infarction is low (~1% at 1 month), and death is generally not due to direct neurological sequelae of the infarct [14]. For example, patients presenting with certain classical lacunar syndromes, such as pure motor hemiparesis and pure sensitive syndrome, have a better prognosis than those with sensorimotor stroke [14].

Laboratory investigations

The CT scan or MRI may be normal, or it may show a small lesion (<1.5 cm) limited to the territory of a single deep perforator and caused by *in situ* small-artery disease.

Stroke of undetermined etiology

This group consists of patients with incomplete evaluation and patients in whom no cause was found despite adequate investigation. In some classifications, such as TOAST [11], patients with coexisting stroke causes (e.g., ICA stenosis and atrial fibrillation) are also included in this category, whereas, in the LSR [9], these patients are classified under mixed etiologies. These different criteria may explain why the frequency of these infarcts varies from 8% in the LSR to 40% in the NINDS Data Bank [48]. Most of the infarcts in this group have the clinical and radiologic characteristics of embolic infarctions [48]. Another important fraction of this group is made up of patients with large-artery disease, but without significant stenosis, or plaques, or with <50% stenosis being found in the ipsilateral corresponding artery. The classification of these patients as 'atherosclerosis without stenosis', as in the LSR, is more appropriate.

Shortcomings of current classifications

There are several important limitations to all current stroke classifications.

Coexisting causes

Although researchers would like to assign infarcts to a single category, a significant percentage of patients present with stroke with more than one possible cause. In the LSR, of the patients with probable cardioembolic strokes, 11% also had severe stenosis (>50%) proximal to the infarcted territory, while 12% had small-vessel disease [32]. If we also consider patients with mild stenosis, a further 40% of patients would have multiple potential causes of stroke. These figures are not surprising, since some risk factors may be involved in the mechanisms of different pathologic processes. For instance, in addition to being a risk factor for small-vessel disease, hypertension predisposes to atherosclerosis and is a risk factor for cardiac abnormalities. Moreover, with the discovery of new potential mechanisms for stroke, such as patent foramen ovale [49] and coagulation abnormalities [50], the number of patients with coexisting stroke causes will tend to increase.

Undetermined cause

Depending on the classification employed, strokes of undetermined origin may account for 40% of all strokes [11,48]. Since this category probably includes a variety of infarct causes [48], it poses a great problem for stroke studies and may partially explain why single agents, which may only be effective against certain stroke subtypes but are tested on all strokes combined, may appear to have a low efficacy.

Acute stroke phase

Ideally, a stroke classification should work best in the acute stroke phase, when patients are evaluated within the very short therapeutic window of 3–6 hours. Unfortunately, mediocre reliability during the acute stage, when compared to the final diagnosis after laboratory work-up, is the Achilles heel of all classifications. Poor interobserver agreement in terms of the history and physical examination, especially in the very acute stage since clinical signs may evolve, may explain this shortcoming. Ideally, the maximal neurologic deficit should be used to classify the patient, but this is obviously inappropriate in the hyperacute setting, when treatment might be particularly effective. Two studies have shown that, even when combined with early CT findings, a clinical presentation of classical lacunar syndrome (i.e., pure motor hemiparesis or sensorimotor stroke) is of little value in the differential diagnosis of lacunar infarction [51,52]. Using patients enrolled in the ECASS I study (European Cooperative Acute Stroke Study I), the positive predictive value of pure motor hemiparesis and sensorimotor stroke, combined with CT findings, was 36% in the placebo group and 33% in tissue plasminogen activator (tPA)-treated patients [52].

Strict versus broad criteria

In order to improve specificity of classification and lessen the likelihood of patient misclassification, strict and artificial criteria are often used. However, such criteria may decrease sensitivity and increase the frequency of cases of undetermined etiology. For instance, in terms of large-artery disease, some classifications define a stenosis of 70% or greater as significant [9], while others use a lower percentage, such as 50% [10]. Although an increasing degree of stenosis is associated with a higher risk of cerebrovascular events, other features, such as plaque composition and the presence of ulcerations, may influence the risk of embolization. Therefore, a patient with an MCA infarct ipsilateral to a 30%–50% stenosis with an ulcerated plaque in the ICA, and without other risk factors, has more features in common with patients with large-artery disease than with those with strokes of undetermined origin, the group to which he/she would be allocated. On the other hand, other categories, such as lacunar infarction, are sometimes very broadly defined and may encompass different lesions [53]. A lacunar syndrome with an infarct <1.5 cm in diameter on CT or MRI does not necessarily mean that this lesion is caused by lipohyalinosis. It has been suggested that atheroma involving the extracranial [54,55] and intracranial vessels [56,57], cardioembolism [58], arteritis and other diseases [59] may be responsible for infarcts limited to the territory of the deep perforators. In fact, it would be reasonable to use the term 'infarct limited to the deep perforators' as a generic descriptive term and to reserve the term 'lacunar infarction' for those infarcts caused by small-vessel disease and no other potential etiology [53].

Stroke recurrence

Finally, even when patients are correctly classified into a group, specific treatment strategies may not avoid further stroke, since up to 38% of patients with recurrent stroke have a new event with an etiology different from that of the index stroke [60]. A recent follow-up of patients included in the NASCET (North American Symptomatic Carotid Endarterectomy Trial) exemplifies this: 20% of strokes in the territory of a symptomatic, 70%–99% ICA stenosis were unrelated to carotid stenosis.

How can classification be improved?

During the last two decades, there have been significant advances in both the detection of microemboli by TCD and in neuroimaging, such as the development of new MRI techniques, e.g., diffusion-weighted imaging (DWI), perfusion-weighted imaging (PWI), and magnetic resonance angiography (MRA). These are promising tools for improving current classifications, especially in the acute stroke phase.

MRI

DWI shows lacunar lesions, even when the results from conventional MRI techniques (e.g., T2-weighted imaging and fluid attenuation inversion recovery) are negative, thus allowing consistent establishment of infarct subtype. In a recent study, the accuracy of DWI in the recognition of acute subcortical infarction, and in differentiating it from nonacute subcortical infarction, was 95%. In addition, although many patients had more than one lesion on conventional MRI, DWI identified the acute lesion in all cases [62]. DWI is well suited to the detection of small acute infarcts, being significantly better than conventional techniques when the lesion is <10 mm [63]. In addition to establishing infarct subtype, DWI can also result in the infarct subtype being reclassified. In a study by Ay et al. [58], in which patients admitted with well-defined classic lacunar syndrome were investigated using DWI, almost one in every six patients had multiple infarctions that were only visible with DWI. The cause of stroke in these patients was reclassified from small-vessel disease to cardioembolism in the light of these new, more accurate findings [58].

Moreover, certain DWI findings strongly suggest the etiology of the infarct, thus directing the clinical work-up and treatment of the patient. Multiple brain infarcts on DWI are relatively common and are suggestive of emboli either from the neck vessels, the heart, or aortic arch [64–67]. Bilateral lesions, or simultaneous lesions in the anterior or posterior circulation, are associated with cardioembolism or hemorheologic abnormalities (e.g., elevated fibrinogen or hematocrit) [65,66].

Another study addressed the diagnostic utility of the combination of MRA and DWI in subtype classification of acute stroke [68]. Using the TOAST criteria, the match between the final diagnosis of infarct subtypes and clinical findings combined with CT or conventional MRI criteria was only 48%, but increased to 56% with MRA alone, 83% with DWI alone, and 94% after DWI plus MRA. In another study, DWI demonstrated the symptomatic lesion to be in a different vascular territory than that suspected clinically or by conventional MRI in 18% of cases, and showed multiple acute lesions in more than one vascular territory in 13% [69]. Furthermore, the combination of DWI and PWI may help in differentiating between embolic and hemodynamic infarctions in internal carotid disease [70].

Doppler ultrasonography

Circulating cerebral emboli can be detected by TCD [71]. The demonstration of cerebral microemboli by TCD in acute cerebral ischemia provides evidence that embolic material is entering the brain, which indirectly suggests that the etiology may also be embolic. Several studies have addressed the role of TCD monitoring of acute stroke patients in the classification of infarct subtype [72–78]. Microemboli were more prevalent in patients with embolic sources (carotid stenosis and cardiac sources) and were only rarely detected in patients with lacunar infarction (**Table 4**). However, great discrepancies were found in the studies, which may be explained by the different definitions of signals specifying

Year	N	Inadequate window (%)	LAD (%)	Cardioembolic (%)	Lacunar (%)	Uncertain (%)	Ref
1994	45	9	87.5	75	0	81.2	72
1995	38	NR	17	17	0	NR	73
1996	280	NR	14.2	NR	4.5	NR	74
1997	90	16	56	33	0	11	75
1997	100	14	61.7	45	NR	40	76
1999	119	16	50	4.5	0	10.3	77
2000	120	23	14.3	52.6	17.6	16.7	78

LAD: large-artery disease; N: number of patients; NR: not reported.

Table 4. Percentage of patients in whom cerebral infarction subtype was related to microemboli.

microemboli, the duration of insonation of the vessels, and the time from stroke onset to TCD examination.

Bilateral TCD monitoring may help to elucidate the origin of emboli. One study showed that ipsilateral microembolic signals occur more frequently in patients with large-artery disease, whereas bilateral signals are suggestive of cardioembolism [78]. The link between microemboli and evidence that embolic material is entering the brain is supported by results demonstrating that microembolic signals detected by TCD are associated with asymptomatic abnormalities in DWI [79]. Nevertheless, there are still shortcomings to TCD monitoring: a significant percentage of patients do not have a suitable temporal bone window to allow monitoring for 30–60 minutes, are too restless, or do not tolerate the device used to fix the probe in place, the signals may represent artifacts or solid or gaseous emboli, and the diverse criteria for monitoring lead to conflicting results. However, developments in the identification of the nature of emboli [80] and consensus on microembolus detection may resolve some of these uncertainties [81].

Conclusion

Stroke classification is of paramount importance not only in providing a common means of communication between investigators, but also for the performance of observational studies and clinical trials. Moreover, a good classification also helps the clinician who wants to incorporate the results of clinical trials into his individual patient management. Without doubt, current classifications have advanced since the 'plugs and leaks' era. However, future classifications should incorporate data obtained from technologic advancements, such as new MRI techniques, especially DWI, and TCD [82,83].

The identification of new risk factors for cerebrovascular disease may reduce the number of strokes with unknown causes, while the use of recently developed methods may reveal the actual cause when multiple potential causes coexist.

References

1. Fields WS. Historical introduction. In: Ginsberg MD, Bogousslavsky J, editors, *Cerebrovascular disease: pathophysiology, diagnosis, and management.* Massachusetts: Blackwell Science, 1998:837–3.

2. Fisher CM. Occlusions of the carotid arteries. *Arch Neurol Psychiatry* 1954;72:187–204.

3. Fisher CM, Curry HB. Pure motor of hemiplegia of vascular origin. *Arch Neurol* 1965;13:30–44.

4. Fisher CM. The arterial lesions underlying lacunes. *Acta Neuropathol (Berlin)* 1969;12:1–15.

5. Besson G, Hommel M. Historical aspects of lacunes and the "lacunar controversy". *Adv Neurol* 1993;62:1–10.

6. Advisory Council for the National Institute of Neurological Diseases and Blindness. A classification and outline of cerebrovascular diseases. *Neurology* 1958;8:395–434.

7. Whisnant JP, Fitzgibbons JP, Kurland LT et al. Natural history of stroke in Rochester, Minnesota, 1945 through 1954. *Stroke* 1971;2:11–22.

8. Mohr JP, Caplan LR, Melski JW et al. The Harvard Cooperative Stroke Study: a prospective registry. *Neurology* 1978;28:754–62.

9. Bogousslavsky J, Van Melle LG, Regli F. The Lausanne Stroke Registry: analysis of 1000 consecutive patients with first stroke. *Stroke* 1988;19:1083–92.

10. Bamford J, Sandercock P, Dennis M et al. Classification and natural history of clinically identifiable subtypes of cerebral infarction. *Lancet* 1991; 337:1521–6.

11. Adams HP Jr, Bendixen BH, Kappelle LJ, and the TOAST investigators. Classification of subtype of acute ischemic stroke: definitions for use in a multicenter clinical trial. *Stroke* 1993;24:34–51.

12. Bamford J. Classifying the mechanisms of ischemic stroke. *Stroke* 2001;32:1096–7.

13. Bamford J, Sandercock P, Dennis M et al. A prospective study of acute cerebrovascular disease in the community: the Oxfordshire Community Stroke Project – 1981-86. 2. Incidence, case fatality rates and overall outcome at one year of cerebral infarction, primary intracerebral hemorrhage and subarachnoid hemorrhage. *J Neurol Neurosurg Psychiatry* 1990:53:16–22.

14. Bamford J, Sandercock P, Jones L et al. The natural history of lacunar infarction: the Oxfordshire Community Stroke Project. *Stroke* 1987; 18:545–51.

15. Petty GW, Brown RD, Whisnant JP et al. Ischemic stroke subtypes: a population-based study of functional outcome, survival, and recurrence. *Stroke* 2000;31:1062–8.

16. The National Institute of Neurological Disorders and Stroke rt-PA Stroke Study Group. Tissue plasminogen activator for acute ischemic stroke. *N Eng J Med* 1995;333:1581–7.

17. The NINDS t-PA Stroke Study Group. Generalized efficacy of t-PA for acute stroke: subgroup analysis of the NINDS t-PA Stroke Trial. *Stroke* 1997;28:2119–25.

18. Barnett HJM, Taylor WD, Eliasziw M et al. Benefit of endarterectomy in patients with symptomatic moderate or severe stenosis. *N Eng J Med* 1998;339:1415–25.

19. Furlan A, Higashida R, Wechsler L et al. Intra-arterial prourokinase for acute ischemic stroke: the PROACT II study: a randomized controlled trial. *JAMA* 1999;282:2003–11.

20. Caplan LR, Mohr JP, Kistler JP et al. Should thrombolytic therapy be the first-line treatment for acute stroke? Thrombolysis – not a panacea for ischemic stroke. *N Eng J Med* 1997;337:1309–10.

21. Grotta J. t-PA – the best current option for most patients. *N Eng J Med* 1997;337:1310–3.

22. Allen CMC. Clinical diagnosis of the acute stroke syndrome. *Q J Med* 1983;52:515–23.

23. Panzer RJ, Feibel JH, Barker WH et al. Predicting the likelihood of hemorrhage in patients with stroke. *Arch Int Med* 1985;145:1800–3.

24. Poungvarin N, Viriyavejakul A, Komontri C. Siriraj stroke score and validation study to distinguish supratentorial intracerebral haemorrhage from infarction. *BMJ* 1991;302:1565–7.

25. Besson G, Robert C, Hommel M et al. Is it clinically possible to distinguish nonhemorrhagic infarct from hemorrhagic stroke? *Stroke* 1995;26:1205–9.

26. Celani MG, Righetti E, Migliacci R et al. Comparability and validity of two clinical scores in the early differential diagnosis of acute stroke. *BMJ* 1994;308:1674–6.

27. Weir CJ, Murray GD, Adams FG et al. Poor accuracy of stroke scoring systems for differential clinical diagnosis of intracranial hemorrhage and infarction. *Lancet* 1994;344:999–1002.

28. Lindley RI, Warlow CP, Wardlaw JM et al. Interobserver reliability of a clinical classification of acute cerebral infarction. *Stroke* 1993;24:1801–4.

29. Madden KP, Karanjia PN, Adams HP Jr et al. Accuracy of initial stroke subtype diagnosis in the TOAST study. *Neurology* 1995:45:1975–9.

30. Caplan LR, Hier DB, D'Cruz I. Cerebral embolism in the Michael Reese Stroke Registry. *Stroke* 1983;14:530–6.

31. Whisnant JP, Basford JR, Bernstein EF. Classification of cerebrovascular diseases III. *Stroke* 1990;21:637–76.

32. Bogousslavsky J, Cachin C, Regli F et al. Cardiac sources of embolism and cerebral infarction – clinical consequences and vascular concomitants: the Lausanne Stroke Registry. *Neurology* 1991;41:855–9.

33. Kittner SJ, Sharkness CM, Sloan MA et al. Infarcts with a cardiac source of embolism in the NINDS Stroke Data Bank: neurologic examination. *Neurology* 1992;42:299–302.

34. Ringelstein EB, Koschorke S, Holling A et al. Computed tomographic patterns of proven embolic brain infarctions. *Ann Neurol* 1989;26:759–65.

35. Kannel WB, Dawber TR, Cohen ME et al. Vascular diseases of the brain - epidemiologic aspects: the Framingham Study. *Am J Public Health* 1965;55:1355–66.

36. Gorelick PB, Caplan LR, Hier DB et al. Racial differences in the distribution of anterior circulation occlusive disease. *Neurology* 1984;34:54–9.

37. Tsiskaridze A, Devuyst G, de Freitas GR et al. Stroke with carotid artery stenosis. *Arch Neurol* 2001;58:605–9.

38. Ringelstein EB, Zeumer H, Angelou D. The pathogenesis of strokes from internal carotid artery occlusion. Diagnostic and therapeutical implications. *Stroke* 1983;14:867–75.

39. Torvik A. The pathogenesis of watershed infarcts in the brain. *Stroke* 1984;15:221–3.

40. Bogousslavsky J, Regli F. Unilateral watershed cerebral infarction. *Neurology* 1986;36:373–7.

41. Bogousslavsky J, Regli F. Borderzone infarctions distal to internal carotid artery occlusion: prognostic implications. *Ann Neurol* 1986;20:346–50.

42. Caplan LR, Hennerici M. Impaired clearance of emboli (washout) is an important link between hypoperfusion, embolism, and ischemic stroke. *Arch Neurol* 1998;55:1475–82.

43. Howard R, Trend P, Russell RWR. Clinical features of ischemia in cerebral arterial border zones after periods of reduced cerebral blood flow. *Arch Neurol* 1987;44:934–40.

44. Bogousslavsky J, Van Melle G, Regli F. Middle cerebral artery pial territory: a study of the Lausanne Stroke Registry. *Ann Neurol* 1989;25:555–60.

45. Fisher CM. Lacunar strokes and infarcts: a review. *Neurology* 1982;32:871–6.

46. Mohr JP. Lacunes. *Stroke* 1982;13:3–11.

47. Fisher CM. Lacunar infarcts. A review. *Cerebrovasc Dis* 1991;1:311–20.

48. Sacco RL, Ellenberg JH, Mohr JP et al. Infarcts of undetermined cause: the NINCDS Stroke Data Bank. *Ann Neurol* 1989;25:382–90.

49. Lechat P, Mas JL, Lascault G et al. Prevalence of patent foramen ovale in patients with stroke. *N Eng J Med* 1988;318:1148–52.

50. Levine SR, Kim S, Deegan MJ et al. Ischemic stroke associated with anti-cardiolipin antibodies. *Stroke* 1987;18:1101–6.

51. Toni D, Del Duca R, Fiorelli M et al. Pure motor hemiparesis and sensorimotor stroke: accuracy of very early clinical diagnosis of lacunar strokes. *Stroke* 1994;25:92–6.

52. Toni D, Iweins F, van Kummer R et al. Identification of lacunar infarcts before thrombolysis in the ECASS I study. *Neurology* 2000;54:684–8.

53. Bogousslavsky J. The plurality of subcortical infarction. *Stroke* 1992;23:629–31.

54. Ghika J, Bogousslavsky J, Regli F. Infarcts in the territory of the deep perforators from the carotid system. *Neurology* 1989;39:507–12.

55. Inzitari D, Eliasziw M, Sharpe BL et al. for the North American Symptomatic Carotid Endarterectomy Trial Group. Risk factors and outcomes of patients with carotid artery stenosis presenting with lacunar stroke. *Neurology* 2000;54:660–6.

56. Fisher CM, Caplan LR. Basilar artery branch occlusion: a cause of pontine infarction. *Neurology* 1971;21:900–5.

57. Bogousslavsky J, Regli F, Maeder P. Intracranial large-artery disease and 'lacunar' infarction. *Cerebrovasc Dis* 1991;1:154–9.

58. Ay H, Oliveira-Filho J, Buonanno FS et al. Diffusion-weighted imaging identifies a subset of lacunar infarction associated with embolic source. *Stroke* 1999;30:2644–50.

59. Lammie GA, Brannan F, Slattery J et al. Nonhypertensive cerebral small-vessel disease: an autopsy study. *Stroke* 1997;28:2222–9.

60. Yamamoto H, Bogousslavsky J. Mechanism of second and further strokes. *J Neurol Neurosurg Psychiatry* 1998;64:771–6.

61. Barnett HJM, Gunton RW, Eliasziw M et al. Causes and severity of ischemic strokes in patients with internal carotid artery stenosis. *JAMA* 2000;283:1429–36.

62. Singer MB, Chong J, Lu D et al. Diffusion-weighted MRI in acute subcortical infarction. *Stroke* 1998;29:133–6.

63. Oliveira-Filho J, Ay H, Schaefer P et al. Diffusion-weighted magnetic resonance imaging identifies the "clinically relevant" small-penetrator infarcts. *Arch Neurol* 2000;57:1009–14.

64. Altieri M, Metz RJ, Müller C et al. Multiple brain infarcts: clinical and neuroimaging patterns using diffusion-weighted magnetic resonance. *Eur Neurol* 1999;42:76–82.

65. Roh JK, Kang DW, Lee SH et al. Significance of multiple brain infarction on diffusion-weighted imaging. *Stroke* 2000;31:688–94.

66. Baird AE, Lovblad KO, Schlaug G et al. Multiple acute stroke syndrome: marker of embolic disease? *Neurology* 2000;54:674–8.

67. Koennecke H-C, Bernarding J, Braun J et al. Scattered brain infarct pattern on diffusion–weighted magnetic resonance imaging in patients with acute ischemic stroke. *Cerebrovasc Dis* 2001;11:157–63.

68. Lee LJ, Kidwell CS, Alger J et al. Impact on stroke subtype diagnosis of early diffusion–weighted magnetic resonance imaging and magnetic resonance angiography. *Stroke* 2000;31:1081–9.

69. Albers GW, Lansberg MG, Norbash AM et al. Yield of diffusion-weighted MRI for detection of potentially relevant findings in stroke patients. *Neurology* 2000;54:1562–7.

70. Szabo K, Kern R, Gass A et al. Acute stroke patterns in patients with internal carotid artery disease: a diffusion-weighted magnetic resonance imaging study. *Stroke* 2001;32:1323–9.

71. Easton JD. Cerebral embolism and Doppler ultrasound. *Cerebrovasc Dis* 1999;9:188–92.

72. Grosset DG, Georgiadis D, Abdullah I et al. Doppler emboli signals vary according to stroke subtype. *Stroke* 1994;25:382–4.

73. Tong DC, Albers GW. Transcranial Doppler-detected microemboli in patients with acute stroke. *Stroke* 1995;26:1588–92.

74. Daffertshofer M, Ries S, Schminke U et al. High-intensity transient signals in patients with cerebral ischemia. *Stroke* 1996;27:1844–9.

75. Del Sette M, Angeli S, Stara I et al. Microembolic signals with serial transcranial Doppler monitoring in acute focal ischemic deficit: a local phenomenon? *Stroke* 1997;28:1311–3.

76. Sliwka U, Lingnau A, Stohlmann W-D et al. Prevalence and time course of microembolic signals in patients with acute stroke. *Stroke* 1997;28:358–63.

77. Kaposzta Z, Young E, Bath PMW et al. Clinical application of asymptomatic embolic signal detection in acute stroke: a prospective study. *Stroke* 1999;30:1814–8.

78. Lund C, Rygh J, Stensrod B et al. Cerebral microembolus detection in an unselected acute ischemic stroke population. *Cerebrovasc Dis* 2000;10:403–8.

79. Kimura K, Minematsu K, Koga M et al. Microembolic signals and diffusion-weighted MR imaging abnormalities in acute ischemic stroke. *AJNR Am J Neuroradiol* 2001;22:1037–42.

80. Devuyst G, Darbellay GA, Vesin J-M et al. Automatic classification of HITS into artifacts or solid or gaseous emboli by a wavelet representation combined with dual–gate TCD. *Stroke* 2001;32:2803–9.

81. Ringelstein EB, Droste DW, Babikian V et al. Consensus on microembolus detection by TCD. *Stroke* 1998;29:725–9.

82. Schwartz A, Gass A, Hennerici MG. Is there a need to reclassify acute stroke patients? *Cerebrovasc Dis* 1998;8(Suppl 1):9–16.

83. Hennerici MG, Schwartz A, Gass A. Acute stroke subtypes - Is there a need for reclassification? *Cerebrovasc Dis* 1998;8(Suppl 2):17–22.

2

CT in acute stroke

Thomas Kucinski, Christoph Koch, & Hermann Zeumer

Introduction

Cranial computed tomography (CT) is the diagnostic technique of choice for patients presenting with acute stroke symptoms due to its ubiquitous availability (even in community hospitals 24 hours a day), practicability in severely impaired patients, and its high sensitivity and specificity in hemorrhage detection [1–3]. Noncontrast CT-scanning allows surveillance of emergency therapeutic approaches such as evacuation of intracerebral hemorrhage (ICH) and thrombolysis in ischemic stroke after exclusion of major early signs of ischemia. Advanced techniques such as CT-angiography (CTA) and CT-perfusion (CTP) can add important etiologic aspects to diagnosis and initial treatment.

This chapter deals with different findings in acute stroke patients with reference to the underlying vascular pathology and the important technical aspects of CT imaging.

Acute hemorrhagic stroke

Primary ICH is the underlying cause of up to 20% of all acute stroke cases, and 5% are due to subarachnoid hemorrhages (SAH) [4]. The importance of CT scanning in stroke patients derives from the difficulty of distinguishing hemorrhagic from ischemic stroke solely on the basis of clinical criteria [5,6]. Usually, standard native CT scans suffice for the initial diagnosis without extensive adjustment of scanning parameters.

Hypertensive bleeding

Most spontaneous hemorrhages occur through disruption of small arteries of the thalamus and putamen [7], caused by vessel wall injury in patients with arterial hypertension. These hemorrhages are typically located either within the basal ganglia (see **Figure 1**), or within the pons, depending on the distribution of long

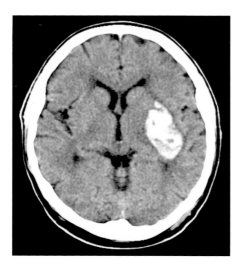

Figure 1. Typical appearance of an acute hypertensive bleed located within the basal ganglia.

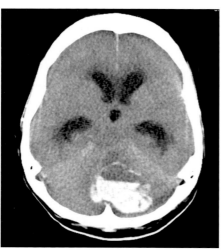

Figure 2. Cerebellar hemorrhage due to anticoagulation during hemofiltration. A horizontal interface divides the hyperdense part (clot) at the bottom from the noncoagulated, nearly isodense blood. Note the compression of the fourth ventricle and aqueduct that has caused hydrocephalus. The global density approximation between white and gray matter is caused by hypoxic ischemic injury.

perforating arteries [8]. They are often accompanied by intraventricular hemorrhage due to their proximity to the ependyma.

Appearance

On cranial CT scans, an acute ICH of any kind usually appears hyperdense compared to the surrounding brain tissue. This is due to a high hematocrit (90%) within the hematoma after clotting and retraction, and the high density of the protein component of hemoglobin. In patients with hemoglobin concentrations <8 g/dL, acute hemorrhage may appear isodense [9]. This phenomenon is also observed in ongoing bleeds or in patients with coagulopathy, in which noncoagulated blood builds isodense compartments within the clot and horizontal clot/blood interfaces can be seen (see **Figure 2**).

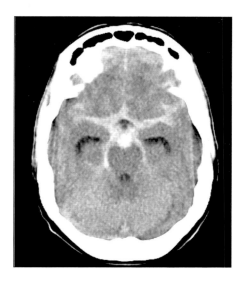

Figure 3. Symmetric subarachnoid hemorrhage within the basal cisterns 4 hours after sudden onset of headache. An aneurysm of the left middle cerebral artery was found on angiography.

In contrast to acute ischemic infarction, mass effect of the hematoma is always present. An extended hypodense ring surrounding the ICH indicating perifocal edema is rarely seen within the first 6 hours after onset of ICH. Not only is an intravenous contrast medium usually unnecessary for correct interpretation but it can also lead to a false diagnosis of tumor lesions in late stages after lysis of the hyperdense clot. MRI details the diagnosis by identifying blood degradation components. Nevertheless, extravasation of contrast media in the acute stage may predict poor outcome [10].

If localization and shape of the hemorrhage do not correlate with the patient's clinical history, other causes of ICH (e.g., arteriovenous (AV) malformations (AVMs), aneurysms, AV fistulae, venous thrombosis, vasculitis, trauma, or amyloid angiopathy [11]) should be considered and evaluated by angiography.

Subarachnoid hemorrhage
Spontaneous rupture of an aneurysm of the basal cerebral arteries, resulting in hemorrhage into the subarachnoid space, may mimic symptoms of acute ischemic stroke leading to incorrect diagnosis, despite the fact that the symptoms of SAH are well described [12]. SAH rarely occurs in combination with AVMs such as dural AV fistulae [13–15].

Appearance
Noncontrast CT scans detect even small amounts of subarachnoid blood, with the overall sensitivity being 92%–98% within the first 24 hours after SAH (see **Figure 3**) [16,17]. Fluid-attenuated inversion-recovery (FLAIR) MRI may prove superior in chronic stages of SAH [18–20], but in an acute emergency session CT

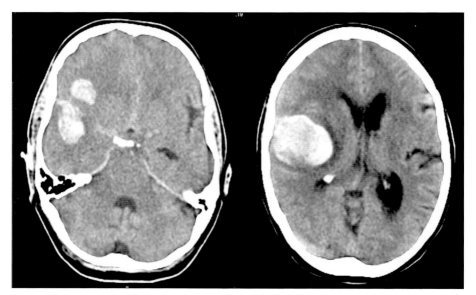

Figure 4. Intracerebral hematoma in a patient 2.5 hours after onset of hemiparesis. Only negligible subarachnoid blood is visible within the basal cisterns, but the proximity to the Sylvian fissure suggests a rupture of an aneurysm of the right middle cerebral artery as the cause for bleeding. This was confirmed by angiography.

is likely to remain the gold standard for the coming years, due to the typical, unmistakable appearance of CT images. SAH localization does not necessarily aid prediction of the origin of the underlying aneurysm [21], except in combination with an intracerebral hematoma, which can be misleading if the ICH is large and an aneurysm rupture is not considered (see **Figure 4**).

Acute ischemic stroke

Most acute ischemic strokes result from thromboembolic occlusion of intracranial arteries. Depending on the occlusion site, various cerebral infarct patterns can be identified in the early and late stages on noncontrast CT scans. In the acute stage, an intravenous contrast medium injection is used to reveal intracranial vessel occlusion by means of CTA, and perfusion deficits by means of CTP.

Anterior cerebral artery territory

Isolated infarction of the anterior cerebral artery (ACA) is rare [22] and local angiopathies such as vasculitis should always be considered if this occurs [23]. ACA infarcts are more frequently found in carotid T-occlusions or following multiple cardioembolic events. When searching for early ischemic findings on CT scans, one should look out for slight hypodensities in frontoparietal brain areas next to the interhemispheric fissure, which represents the characteristic territory. Early

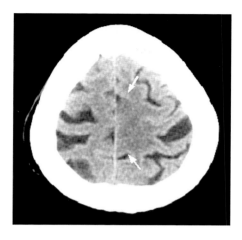

Figure 5. A small, hypodense cortical area 3 hours after symptom onset indicates early ischemic alterations within the anterior cerebral artery territory. Identification of this lesion is only possible because of the adjacent, apparently normal, cortical rim on the contralateral side.

changes in acute ischemic stroke are clearly visible when comparing the cortical rim with the adjacent contralateral cortex (see **Figure 5**). Otherwise, they may easily be missed, which may result in an underestimation of early hypodensities before thrombolytic therapy, e.g., in carotid T-occlusion. There are no diagnostic difficulties in later stages (after 6–12 hours) of ACA infarctions due to progressive development of clear hypodensities and subsequent increasing tissue contrast compared with normal brain tissue.

Middle cerebral artery territory

About 75% of all ischemic events involve the middle cerebral artery (MCA) territory, hence it receives the greatest assignment of acute stroke imaging [24]. Symptoms of MCA acute ischemic stroke vary between minor sensorial or motor deficits and major symptoms such as aphasia, hemiplegia, and enforced head and gaze deviation combined with mild impaired consciousness. Due to recent developments in intra-arterial [25–30] and systemic thrombolysis [31–35], more patients are being scanned earlier to rule out initial hemorrhage and large, extended brain tissue changes that may increase the rate of symptomatic bleedings from thrombolysis. In all such cases, a careful analysis of early ischemic alterations on native CT scans is recommended [36,37].

The hyperdense MCA sign

A blood clot in the MCA is visible as a hyperdense middle cerebral artery sign (HMCAS) [38–40], and is most evident along the horizontal part of the MCA lying within the image plane (see **Figure 6**). It appears as a vessel segment of higher density than other parts of the same vessel, the contralateral MCA, and the basilar artery. Even though the HMCAS has been associated with a more severe stroke course [41–43], it is not an unequivocal sign of an occlusion of the MCA and does not represent ischemic changes in brain parenchyma. Consequently its prognostic

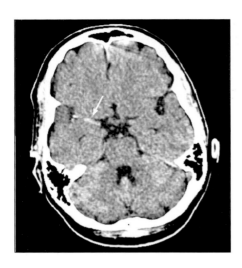

Figure 6. Hyperdense middle cerebral artery sign 1 hour 45 minutes after stroke onset.

value—which is adversely affected by low sensitivity [44,45], low negative predictive value [41], and false positive results due to high hematocrit and vessel wall calcifications [46]—is not comparable with the prognostic value achieved by observation of changes in tissue attenuation [43].

Posterior cerebral artery territory

Occlusions of the posterior cerebral artery (PCA) cause infarctions in occipital and temporal brain tissue to a varying degree [47]. Proximal occlusions result in infarctions of the occipital lobe and the temporobasal parenchyma, including the posterolateral periventricular region and the dorsolateral thalamus [48] if the posterior choroidal [49] or thalamo-perforating arteries are affected (see **Figure 7**). Distally located occlusions are followed by smaller infarcts, often involving the calcarine fissure. In the first hours after stroke onset, these infarcts may be overlooked in CT if clinical information is lacking or misleading [50]. A further hindrance to early diagnosis results from the proximity to bony structures. Because of this, such signs in the PCA territory are rarely detected early and in most infarcts are only seen in later stages.

Territorial infarcts: early signs of cerebral infarction

The typical appearance of an infarction due to thromboembolic occlusion of an intracranial artery is a clearly delineated, wedge-shaped hypodense area involving both the cerebral cortex and the adjacent white matter (see **Figure 8**). The distribution of these lesions is closely related to the territory supplied by the affected artery. Hemorrhagic transformation is rarely seen within the first 24 hours, but occurs in more than 40% of all territorial infarctions in the subacute stage [51,52].

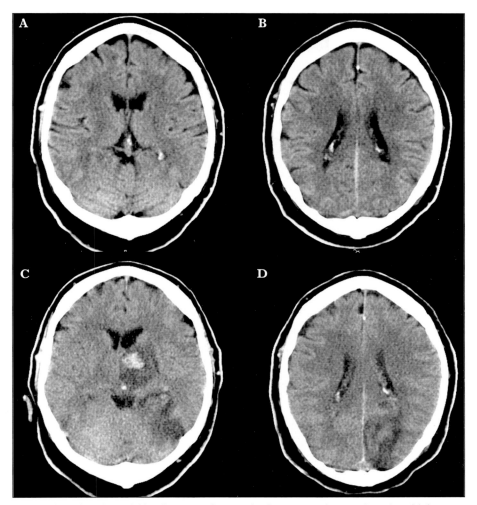

Figure 7. Infarction within the posterior cerebral artery and posterior choroidal artery territory (C and D) with hemorrhagic transformation one day after stroke onset. The initial CT 4 hours after symptom onset (A and B) does not reveal substantial early changes. Only after comparison with the follow-up CT can a localized sulcal effacement and minimal hypodensity of the mesial occipital lobe be noticed.

Hypodensity of the lentiform nucleus is always found following proximal occlusion of the MCA within the sphenoid segment [53]. This is caused by the occlusion of the lenticulostriate arteries, which are functionally noncollateralized terminal arteries. In contrast, the extent of cortical MCA-territory ischemia is dependent on the sufficiency of leptomeningeal anastomoses from the ACA and PCA and on the degree of early reperfusion of the brain region in which the collateral blood supply allows functional recovery of impaired neurons (penumbra) [54–58].

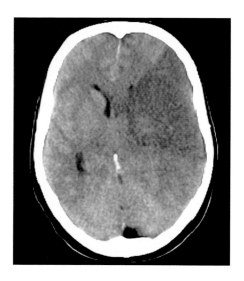

Figure 8. Depiction of an infarction of the left middle cerebral artery territory on a CT scan ~24 hours after stroke onset. A wedge-shaped, well-delineated area of hypodense infarcted tissue is visible, affecting the cortex, adjacent white matter, and basal ganglia. Subtle isodensity within the infarction represents minor hemorrhagic transformation. A considerable space-occupying effect due to edematous swelling gives rise to substantial midline shift.

Hypodensity on CT

Hypodensities are visible on CT scans because of elevated water content in the ischemic tissue due to a primarily cytotoxic, secondarily vasogenic, edema [59]. This increases the volume of brain tissue and leads to hemispheric swelling, mostly evident within the first 3–10 days. Within this time period, the first maximum of hypodensity is reached followed by a phase of near isodensity in comparison to the surrounding viable tissue—the so-called 'fogging stage' [60]. After resorption of necrotic tissue, a hypodense defect is seen consisting of glial scars and cerebrospinal fluid; this is the final stage of the infarct [61].

The development of early hypodensities can be monitored using sequential CT scans beginning as early as 6 hours after onset of symptoms [62], although subtle changes can be observed as early as 45 minutes after symptom onset [63]. This is due to a drop in tissue attenuation by about 1.5 Hounsfield units (HU) for each percent increase of water content [64], which is substantially lower than previously assumed [65]. At the beginning of the drop in tissue attenuation, the margins of the lentiform nucleus are surrounded by well-defined, hypodense, white matter structures. Gradually, these margins vanish due to density approximation between gray matter and the inner and outer capsule (see **Figure 9**) [66–68]. This phenomenon can also be observed in superficial gray matter, and can be better seen in tissue surrounding the Sylvian fissure [67,69], where gray matter on either side of the fissure is close together (see **Figure 10**). The lobular cortical ribbon eventually fades ('loss of the insular ribbon'), accompanied by an effacement of adjacent cerebral sulci (see **Figure 11**) [44,66,70,71]. These gradual changes must be carefully judged, and, depending on the clinical presentation, always compared with presumably unaffected gray matter on either the contralateral or

anterior inferior cerebellar artery show great variability due to varying collateralization by the PICA [100,101]. They almost always involve the inferior anterolateral regions of the cerebellum and the peduncle, but a distinct differentiation between a territorial and a hemodynamic pattern in these infarctions is often impossible [99].

Brain ischemia: early signs

Early signs of brain ischemia are detectable in gray matter as opposed to white matter. This may be due to the fact that CT fails to differentiate subtle hypodensities in white matter. Another explanation is the predominance of early water uptake in gray matter, which has a different cytoarchitecture to white matter [102].

MR diffusion imaging is more sensitive to early changes in ischemic brain tissue [103] since it detects the decrease in free diffusible water: ion pump failure leads to the movement of water molecules from the extracellular space to the intracellular space [104]. Unlike MR diffusion imaging, CT is only sensitive to the net uptake of water in brain tissue, irrespective of its location [105]. Consequently, diffusion impairment has been found to be reversible in early reperfused tissue [76,106–108], in contrast to early hypodensities found by CT, which have never appeared to be reversible in acute thromboembolic ischemia [109,110]. Visible early CT hypodensities occur later than diffusion impairment [64] and probably represent the core of ischemia with the most severe reduction of cerebral blood flow. Thus, hypodensity visualized using CT delineates the area of subsequent infarction, while diffusion impairment as visualized by early MR diffusion imaging may indicate reversible ischemia as well as irreversible infarction.

The prognostic value of early CT changes

Von Kummer et al. [70,110,111] reported that early hypodensities could be used to predict unfavorable outcome in thrombolytic therapy if they exceeded one third of the MCA territory and were thus related to large infarctions and substantial hemorrhage [35,112]. The exclusion of such patients from thrombolysis with recombinant tissue plasminogen activator (rtPA), even within 3 hours after stroke, was recommended [33,113]. Other studies have shown a high likelihood of poor outcome if hypodensity exceeds 50% of MCA-territory [44,114,115], which is not surprising since hypodensity represents infarcted tissue.

Future studies on thrombolytic therapy are necessary to clarify whether or not diffusion imaging has an equally dependable prognostic value [116]. However, the higher contrast of early ischemic lesions in diffusion-weighted imaging

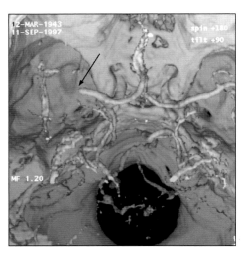

Figure 16. CT-angiography (shaded-surface display) of an acute occlusion of the middle cerebral artery trunk (arrow).

compared with CT [64,117–121] and the possibility of multislice perfusion studies will substantially increase the role of MRI in stroke imaging in the future [122–125].

The great disadvantage of the early application of CT in cerebral ischemia is its high dependency on interpretation coupled with the technical insufficiency of CT studies and the lack of training of physicians [126–128]. Training in CT interpretation has already resulted in a substantial increase in the number of patients correctly excluded from thrombolysis [129].

The quantification of cortical hypodensity in about one third of the MCA territory has been considered unreliable [37,130], despite earlier studies showing sufficient sensitivity and adequate inter-rater agreement between neuroradiologists [36,71]. Within the first 3 hours of ischemic stroke, early CT signs were not predictive for adverse outcome in the National Institute of Neurologic Disorders and Stroke (NINDS) study population [131], which can be explained by the delay in the formation of conspicuous hypodensities. Relying on the 'one third' criterion, the ECASS II study [34] failed to demonstrate significant clinical benefit based on primary endpoints in patients treated within 6 hours. Therefore, further variables should be considered in thrombolytic treatment within 3 to 6 hours after onset, i.e., CT-perfusion [132,133], a perfusion/diffusion mismatch in MRI (see Chapter 3) [134,135], and the location of the arterial occlusion, as determined by CTA (see Chapter 4) (**Figure 16**) [136–138]. Intracranial occlusion of the ICA bifurcation has been shown to be predictive of fatal outcome in patients selected for local intra-arterial thrombolysis [69]. Future improvements in the selection of patients being considered for thrombolysis can be expected as different approaches to quantification of brain perfusion are developed and used [56,122,123,139–141].

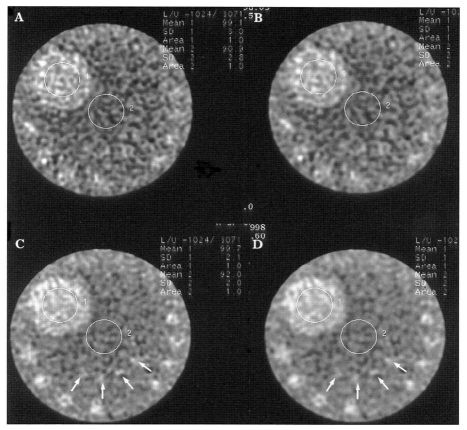

Figure 17. Effect of tube current and image reconstruction algorithm on signal-to-noise ratio in a phantom. Upper row (A and B): tube current 200 mA; lower row (C and D): 400 mA. Left column (A and C): standard kernel; right column (B and D): smoothing kernel. Increasing tube current decreases image noise (i.e., standard deviation of mean density in a region of interest) from (A) 2.8 HU to (C) 2.0 HU. A further decrease is achieved by the smoothing kernel to (B) 2.4 HU and (D) 1.7 HU, respectively. Delineation of small hyperdense areas in C and D is improved substantially or actually made possible (arrows).

Technical aspects

Density resolution

In CT scanning, density resolution is dependent on the detected photon count emanating from the x-ray source, which is required to create the raw data matrix of a CT image. An increase in slice thickness and an increase in tube current both decrease image noise and increase the signal-to-noise ratio (SNR) (**Figure 17**). Helical data acquisition in noncontrast scanning should generally be avoided due to an unfavorable lower contrast resolution and artifacts adjacent to the skull [142].

Slice thickness

Slice thickness should not exceed 8 mm because this leads to inadequate spatial resolution in the z-axis and partial volume effects due to incomplete inclusion of the object within the slice, leading to divergent density values. Fortunately, modern scanners have powerful tubes, which allow fast scanning with sufficient tube currents. Due to beam hardening between petrous bone structures (Hounsfield artifact), special attention must be given to slice thickness in basal regions up to the clinoid process. Tube current should be increased at this point, and slice thickness decreased such that it does not exceed 3 mm. It is important to note that since the radiation dose increases with increased tube current, these specially adjusted scanning parameters should only be used in acute stroke (emergency) patients within the first 6 hours. Volume artifact reduction scanning, i.e., adding several millimetric slices to achieve one thick slice, can decrease Hounsfield artifacts and improve image quality in the posterior fossa.

Signal-to-noise ratio

The chosen image reconstruction algorithm influences the SNR: a smoothing algorithm will increase the SNR at the tolerable expense of a decreased spatial resolution (see **Figure 17**), the resulting in-plane resolution still being four-fold higher than in MRI. A higher image contrast can be achieved with reduced image blurring and allows access to a narrower image window (e.g., center 35, width 45 HU). Increasing the contrast resolution is the goal in the search for small density changes of 2–46 HU within the first hours after acute stroke [143].

Positioning

Proper positioning and head fixation are necessary to avoid oblique scanning in the transverse plane, which may produce misinterpretation on comparison of the hemispheres.

CT-perfusion

Dynamic CT (the scanning of brain tissue during the passage of a bolus of contrast media) was developed early in the CT era [144], but adequate scanner hardware and software has only recently become available to allow practical application [145,146]. Shortly after native CT scanning, the patient's head is positioned according to a predetermined clinically suspicious slice, and fast repeated scans of the same slice are performed during application of a sufficiently high and dense intravenous contrast medium bolus [147]. Extraordinary time resolutions can be realized through continuous data acquisition and segmental reconstruction of serial images of up to 10 images per second. With multislice scanners, more than one slice may be studied simultaneously.

69. Truwit CL, Barkovich AJ, Gean-Marton A et al. Loss of the insular ribbon: Another early CT sign of acute middle cerebral artery infarction. *Radiology* 1990;176(3):801–6.

70. Marks MP, Holmgren EB, Fox AJ et al. Evaluation of early computed tomographic findings in acute ischemic stroke. *Stroke* 1999;30(2):389–92.

71. von Kummer R, Nolte PN, Schnittger H et al. Detectability of cerebral hemisphere ischaemic infarcts by CT within 6 h of stroke. *Neuroradiology* 1996;38(1):31–3.

72. Scott JN, Buchan AM, Sevick RJ. Correlation of neurologic dysfunction with CT findings in early acute stroke. *Can J Neurol Sci* 1999;26(3):182–9.

73. von Kummer R, Allen KL, Holle R et al. Acute stroke: Usefulness of early CT findings before thrombolytic therapy. *Radiology* 1997;205(2):327–33.

74. Stapf C, Hofmeister C, Hartmann A et al. Predictive value of clinical lacunar syndromes for lacunar infarcts on magnetic resonance brain imaging. *Acta Neurol Scand* 2000;101(1):13–8.

75. Toni D, Iweins F, von Kummer R et al. Identification of lacunar infarcts before thrombolysis in the ECASS I study. *Neurology* 2000;54(3):684–8.

76. Doege CA, Kerskens CM, Romero BI et al. MRI of small human stroke shows reversible diffusion changes in subcortical gray matter. *Neuroreport* 2000;11(9):2021–4.

77. Zeumer H, Ringelstein EB, Klose KC. Lacunar infarcts in computerized tomography. Angiographic findings and differential diagnostic viewpoints. *ROFO Fortschr Geb Rontgenstr Nuklearmed* 1981;134(5):488–94.

78. Ringelstein EB, Weiller C. Pattern of cerebral infarct in computerized tomography. Pathophysiologic concepts, validation and clinical relevance. *Nervenarzt* 1990;61(8):462–71.

79. Phillips SJ. Pathogenesis, diagnosis, and treatment of hypertension-associated stroke. *Am J Hypertens* 1989;2(6 Pt 1):493–501.

80. Mull M, Schwarz M, Thron A. Cerebral hemispheric low-flow infarcts in arterial occlusive disease. Lesion patterns and angiomorphological conditions. *Stroke* 1997;28(1):118–23.

81. Ringelstein EB, Zeumer H, Angelou D. The pathogenesis of strokes from internal carotid artery occlusion. Diagnostic and therapeutical implications. *Stroke* 1983;14(6):867–75.

82. Ringelstein EB, Zeumer H, Schneider R. Contribution of computer tomography of the brain to differential typology and differential therapy of ischemic cerebral infarct. *Fortschr Neurol Psychiatr* 1985;53(9):315–36.

83. Bladin CF, Chambers BR. Frequency and pathogenesis of hemodynamic stroke. *Stroke* 1994;25(11):2179–82.

84. Neumann-Haefelin T, Wittsack HJ, Fink GR et al. Diffusion- and perfusion-weighted MRI: influence of severe carotid artery stenosis on the DWI/PWI mismatch in acute stroke. *Stroke* 2000;31(6):1311–7.

85. Ringelstein EB, Zeumer H, Hundgen R et al. Angiologic and prognostic evaluation of brain stem injuries. Clinical, doppler-sonographic and neuroradiological findings. *Dtsch Med Wochenschr* 1983;108(43):1625–31.

86. Kataoka S, Hori A, Shirakawa T et al. Paramedian pontine infarction. Neurological/topographical correlation. *Stroke* 1997;28(4):809–15.

87. Ehsan T, Hayat G, Malkoff MD et al. Hyperdense basilar artery. An early computed tomography sign of thrombosis. *J Neuroimaging* 1994;4(4):200–5.

88. Zeumer H, Hacke W, Ringelstein EB. Local intraarterial thrombolysis in vertebrobasilar thromboembolic disease. *AJNR Am J Neuroradiol* 1983;4(3):401–4.

89. Bruckmann HJ, Ringelstein EB, Buchner H et al. Vascular recanalizing techniques in the hind brain circulation. *Neurosurg Rev* 1987;10(3):197–8.

90. Cross DT, 3rd, Moran CJ, Akins PT et al. Collateral circulation and outcome after basilar artery thrombolysis. *AJNR Am J Neuroradiol* 1998;19(8):1557–63.

91. Brandt T, von Kummer R, Muller-Kuppers M et al. Thrombolytic therapy of acute basilar artery occlusion. Variables affecting recanalization and outcome. *Stroke* 1996;27(5):875–81.

92. Brandt T, Knauth M, Wildermuth S et al. CT angiography and Doppler sonography for emergency assessment in acute basilar artery ischemia. *Stroke* 1999;30(3):606–12.

93. Min WK, Kim YS, Kim JY et al. Atherothrombotic cerebellar infarction: Vascular lesion-MRI correlation of 31 cases. *Stroke* 1999;30(11):2376–81.

94. Graf KJ, Pessin MS, DeWitt LD et al. Proximal intracranial territory posterior circulation infarcts in the New England Medical Center Posterior Circulation Registry. *Eur Neurol* 1997;37(3):157–68.

95. Kim JS, Lee JH, Choi CG. Patterns of lateral medullary infarction: Vascular lesion-magnetic resonance imaging correlation of 34 cases. *Stroke* 1998;29(3):645–52.

96. Sacco RL, Freddo L, Bello JA et al. Wallenberg's lateral medullary syndrome. Clinical-magnetic resonance imaging correlations. *Arch Neurol* 1993;50(6):609–14.

97. Savoiardo M, Bracchi M, Passerini A et al. The vascular territories in the cerebellum and brainstem: CT and MR study. *AJNR Am J Neuroradiol* 1987;8(2):199–209.

98. Malm J, Kristensen B, Carlberg B et al. Clinical features and prognosis in young adults with infratentorial infarcts. *Cerebrovasc Dis* 1999;9(5):282–9.

99. Canaple S, Bogousslavsky J. Multiple large and small cerebellar infarcts. *J Neurol Neurosurg Psychiatry* 1999;66(6):739–45.

100. Roquer J, Lorenzo JL, Pou A. The anterior inferior cerebellar artery infarcts: A clinical-magnetic resonance imaging study. *Acta Neurol Scand* 1998;97(4):225–30.

101. Amarenco P, Rosengart A, DeWitt LD et al. Anterior inferior cerebellar artery territory infarcts. Mechanisms and clinical features. *Arch Neurol* 1993;50(2):154–61.

102. Kuroiwa T, Nagaoka T, Ueki M et al. Different apparent diffusion coefficient: Water content correlations of gray and white matter during early ischemia. *Stroke* 1998;29(4):859–65.

103. Lansberg MG, Albers GW, Beaulieu C et al. Comparison of diffusion-weighted MRI and CT in acute stroke. *Neurology* 2000;54(8):1557–61.

104. Mintorovitch J, Yang GY, Shimizu H et al. Diffusion-weighted magnetic resonance imaging of acute focal cerebral ischemia: Comparison of signal intensity with changes in brain water and Na+,K(+)-ATPase activity. *J Cereb Blood Flow Metab* 1994;14(2):332–6.

105. von Kummer R. CT of acute cerebral ischemia letter. *Radiology* 2000;216(2):611–3.

106. Li F, Liu KF, Silva MD et al. Transient and permanent resolution of ischemic lesions on diffusion-weighted imaging after brief periods of focal ischemia in rats: Correlation with histopathology. *Stroke* 2000;31(4):946–54.

107. Kidwell CS, Saver JL, Mattiello J et al. Thrombolytic reversal of acute human cerebral ischemic injury shown by diffusion/perfusion magnetic resonance imaging. *Ann Neurol* 2000;47(4):462–9.

108. Fiehler J, Foth M, Kucinski T et al. Severe ADC decreases do not predict irreversible tissue damage in humans. *Stroke* 2002;33(1):79–86.

109. Grond M, von Kummer R, Sobesky J et al. Early x-ray hypoattenuation of brain parenchyma indicates extended critical hypoperfusion in acute stroke. *Stroke* 2000;31(1):133–9.

110. von Kummer R, Bourquain H, Bastianello S et al. Early Prediction of Irreversible Brain Damage after Ischemic Stroke at CT. *Radiology* 2001;219(1):95–100.

111. von Kummer R, Weber J. Brain and vascular imaging in acute ischemic stroke: The potential of computed tomography. *Neurology* 1997;49(5 Suppl. 4):52S-55S.

112. Larrue V, von Kummer R, del Zoppo G et al. Hemorrhagic transformation in acute ischemic stroke. Potential contributing factors in the European Cooperative Acute Stroke Study. *Stroke* 1997;28(5):957–60.

113. Adams HP, Jr., Brott TG, Furlan AJ et al. Guidelines for thrombolytic therapy for acute stroke: A supplement to the guidelines for the management of patients with acute ischemic stroke. A statement for healthcare professionals from a Special Writing Group of the Stroke Council, American Heart Association. *Circulation* 1996;94(5):1167–74.

114. Krieger DW, Demchuk AM, Kasner SE et al. Early clinical and radiological predictors of fatal brain swelling in ischemic stroke. *Stroke* 1999;30(2):287–92.

115. Barber PA, Demchuk AM, Zhang J et al. Validity and reliability of a quantitative computed tomography score in predicting outcome of hyperacute stroke before thrombolytic therapy. ASPECTS Study Group. Alberta Stroke Programme Early CT Score published erratum appears in Lancet 2000 Jun 17;355(9221):2170. *Lancet* 2000;355(9216):1670–4.

116. Barber PA, Darby DG, Desmond PM et al. Identification of major ischemic change. Diffusion-weighted imaging versus computed tomography. *Stroke* 1999;30(10):2059–65.

117. Urbach H, Flacke S, Keller E et al. Detectability and detection rate of acute cerebral hemisphere infarcts on CT and diffusion-weighted MRI. *Neuroradiology* 2000;42(10):722–7.

118. Fiebach JB, Schellinger PD, Jansen O et al. CT and diffusion-weighted MR imaging in randomized order: diffusion-weighted imaging results in higher accuracy and lower interrater variability in the diagnosis of hyperacute ischemic stroke. *Stroke* 2002;33(9):2206–10.

119. Fiebach J, Jansen O, Schellinger P et al. Comparison of CT with diffusion-weighted MRI in patients with hyperacute stroke. *Neuroradiology* 2001;43(8):628–32.

120. Lansberg MG, Albers GW, Beaulieu C et al. Comparison of diffusion-weighted MRI and CT in acute stroke. *Neurology* 2000;54(8):1557–61.

121. Gonzalez RG, Schaefer PW, Buonanno FS et al. Diffusion-weighted MR imaging: diagnostic accuracy in patients imaged within 6 hours of stroke symptom onset. *Radiology* 1999;210(1):155–62.

122. Smith AM, Grandin CB, Duprez T et al. Whole brain quantitative CBF, CBV, and MTT measurements using MRI bolus tracking: Implementation and application to data acquired from hyperacute stroke patients. *J Magn Reson Imaging* 2000;12(3):400–10.

123. Neumann Haefelin T, Wittsack HJ, Wenserski F et al. Diffusion- and perfusion-weighted MRI. The DWI/PWI mismatch region in acute stroke. *Stroke* 1999;30(8):1591–7.

124. Schellinger PD, Jansen O, Fiebach JB et al. Monitoring intravenous recombinant tissue plasminogen activator thrombolysis for acute ischemic stroke with diffusion and perfusion MRI. *Stroke* 2000;31(6):1318–28.

125. Warach S. New imaging strategies for patient selection for thrombolytic and neuroprotective therapies. *Neurology* 2001;57(Suppl. 2):S48–S52.

126. Grotta JC, Chiu D, Lu M et al. Agreement and variability in the interpretation of early CT changes in stroke patients qualifying for intravenous rtPA therapy. *Stroke* 1999;30(8):1528–33.

127. Schriger DL, Kalafut M, Starkman S et al. Cranial computed tomography interpretation in acute stroke: Physician accuracy in determining eligibility for thrombolytic therapy. *JAMA* 1998;279(16):1293–7.

128. Cooper RJ, Schriger DL. How accurate is a CT scan in identifying acute strokes? *West J Med* 1999;171:356–7.

129. von Kummer R. Effect of training in reading CT scans on patient selection for ECASS II. *Neurology* 1998;51(3 Suppl. 3):50S–52S.

130. Wardlaw JM, Dorman PJ, Lewis SC et al. Can stroke physicians and neuroradiologists identify signs of early cerebral infarction on CT? *J Neurol Neurosurg Psychiatry* 1999;67(5):651–3.

131. Patel SC, Levine SR, Tilley BC et al. Lack of clinical significance of early ischemic changes on computed tomography in acute stroke. *JAMA* 2001;286(22):2830–8.

132. Kirchhof K, Schramm P, Klotz E et al. The value of multi-slice computed tomography for early diagnosis of focal cerebral ischemia. *Rofo Fortschr Geb Rontgenstr Neuen Bildgeb Verfahr* 2002;174(9):1089–95.

133. Wintermark M, Reichhart M, Cuisenaire O et al. Comparison of admission perfusion computed tomography and qualitative diffusion- and perfusion-weighted magnetic resonance imaging in acute stroke patients. *Stroke* 2002;33(8):2025–31.

134. Schlaug G, Benfield A, Baird AE et al. The ischemic penumbra: operationally defined by diffusion and perfusion MRI. *Neurology* 1999;53(7):1528–37.

135. Albers GW. Advances in intravenous thrombolytic therapy for treatment of acute stroke. *Neurology* 2001;57(Suppl. 2):S77–81.

136. Wildermuth S, Knauth M, Brandt T et al. Role of CT angiography in patient selection for thrombolytic therapy in acute hemispheric stroke. *Stroke* 1998;29(5):935–8.

137. Knauth M, von Kummer R, Jansen O et al. Potential of CT angiography in acute ischemic stroke. *AJNR Am J Neuroradiol* 1997;18(6):1001–10.

138. John C, Elsner E, Muller A et al. Computer tomographic diagnosis of acute cerebral ischemmia. *Radiologe* 1997;37(11):853–9.

139. Heiss WD, Kracht L, Grond M et al. Early (11)C Flumazenil/H(2)O positron emission tomography predicts irreversible ischemic cortical damage in stroke patients receiving acute thrombolytic therapy. *Stroke* 2000;31(2):366–9.

140. Schlaug G, Benfield A, Baird AE et al. The ischemic penumbra: Operationally defined by diffusion and perfusion MRI. *Neurology* 1999;53(7):1528–37.

141. Karonen JO, Vanninen RL, Liu Y et al. Combined diffusion and perfusion MRI with correlation to single-photon emission CT in acute ischemic stroke. Ischemic penumbra predicts infarct growth. *Stroke* 1999;30(8):1583–90.

142. Bahner ML, Reith W, Zuna I et al. Spiral CT vs incremental CT: Is spiral CT superior in imaging of the brain? *Eur Radiol* 1998;8(3):416–20.

143. Lev MH, Farkas J, Gemmete JJ et al. Acute stroke: Improved nonenhanced CT detection — Benefits of soft-copy interpretation by using variable window width and center level settings. *Radiology* 1999;213(1):150–5.

144. Hacker H, Becker H. Time controlled computed tomographic angiography. *J Comput Assist Tomogr* 1977;1(4):405–9.

145. Nabavi DG, Cenic A, Craen RA et al. CT assessment of cerebral perfusion: Experimental validation and initial clinical experience. *Radiology* 1999;213(1):141–9.

146. Cenic A, Nabavi DG, Craen RA et al. Dynamic CT measurement of cerebral blood flow: A validation study. *AJNR Am J Neuroradiol* 1999;20(1):63–73.

147. Hamberg LM, Hunter GJ, Halpern EF et al. Quantitative high-resolution measurement of cerebrovascular physiology with slip-ring CT. *AJNR Am J Neuroradiol* 1996;17(4):639–50.

148. Axel L. Cerebral blood flow determination by rapid-sequence computed tomography: Theoretical analysis. *Radiology* 1980;137(3):679–86.

149. Axel L. A method of calculating brain blood flow with a CT dynamic scanner. *Adv Neurol* 1981;30:67–71.

150. Klotz E, Konig M. Perfusion measurements of the brain: Using dynamic CT for the quantitative assessment of cerebral ischemia in acute stroke. *Eur J Radiol* 1999;30(3):170–84.

151. Konig M, Klotz E, Heuser L. Cerebral perfusion CT: Theoretical aspects, methodical implementation and clinical experience in the diagnosis of ischemic cerebral infarction. *Rofo Fortschr Geb Rontgenstr Neuen Bildgeb Verfahr* 2000;172(3):210–8.

152. Touho H, Karasawa J. Evaluation of time-dependent thresholds of cerebral blood flow and transit time during the acute stage of cerebral embolism: A retrospective study. *Surg Neurol* 1996;46(2):135–45; discussion 145–6.

153. Rother J, Jonetz-Mentzel L, Fiala A et al. Hemodynamic assessment of acute stroke using dynamic single-slice computed tomographic perfusion imaging. *Arch Neurol* 2000;57(8):1161–6.

154. Konig M, Banach-Planchamp R, Kraus M et al. CT perfusion imaging in acute ischemic cerebral infarct: Comparison of cerebral perfusion maps and conventional CT findings. *Rofo Fortschr Geb Rontgenstr Neuen Bildgeb Verfahr* 2000;172(3):219–26.

155. Koenig M, Kraus M, Theek C et al. Quantitative assessment of the ischemic brain by means of perfusion-related parameters derived from perfusion CT. *Stroke* 2001;32(2):431–7.

156. Tatlisumak T. Is CT or MRI the method of choice for imaging patients with acute stroke? Why should men divide if fate has united? *Stroke* 2002;33(9):2144–5.

157. Hamberg LM, Hunter GJ, Kierstead D et al. Measurement of cerebral blood volume with subtraction three-dimensional functional CT. *AJNR Am J Neuroradiol* 1996;17(10):1861–9.

158. Na DG, Byun HS, Lee KH et al. Acute occlusion of the middle cerebral artery: Early evaluation with triphasic helical CT — Preliminary results. *Radiology* 1998;207(1):113–22.

159. Hunter GJ, Hamberg LM, Ponzo JA et al. Assessment of cerebral perfusion and arterial anatomy in hyperacute stroke with three-dimensional functional CT: Early clinical results. *AJNR Am J Neuroradiol* 1998;19(1):29–37.

160. Lee KH, Cho SJ, Byun HS et al. Triphasic perfusion computed tomography in acute middle cerebral artery stroke: A correlation with angiographic findings. *Arch Neurol* 2000;57(7):990–9.

161. Lee KH, Lee SJ, Cho SJ et al. Usefulness of triphasic perfusion computed tomography for intravenous thrombolysis with tissue-type plasminogen activator in acute ischemic stroke. *Arch Neurol* 2000;57(7):1000–8.

162. Meyer JS, Hayman LA, Sakai F et al. High-resolution three-dimensional measurement of localized cerebral blood flow by CT scanning and stable xenon clearance: Effect of cerebral infarction and ischemia. *Trans Am Neurol Assoc* 1979;104:85–9.

163. Firlik AD, Rubin G, Yonas H et al. Relation between cerebral blood flow and neurologic deficit resolution in acute ischemic stroke. *Neurology* 1998;51(1):177–82.

164. Rubin G, Levy EI, Scarrow AM et al. Remote effects of acute ischemic stroke: A xenon CT cerebral blood flow study. *Cerebrovasc Dis* 2000;10(3):221–8.

165. Marchal G, Bouvard G, Iglesias S et al. Predictive value of (99m)Tc-HMPAO-SPECT for neurological Outcome/Recovery at the acute stage of stroke. *Cerebrovasc Dis* 2000;10(1):8–17.

3

MRI in acute stroke

Tobias Neumann-Haefelin & Michael E. Moseley

Introduction

The use of magnetic resonance imaging (MRI) in the acute stroke setting has increased over the past few years due to the unique sensitivity of several new MRI techniques for the rapid detection of cerebral ischemia. These new techniques include diffusion-weighted imaging (DWI), perfusion-weighted imaging (PWI), and high-speed MR-angiography (MRA). They are typically combined in so-called 'integrated MR-exams', which also include T2*-weighted sequences ('bleed screen') and conventional techniques. These scans can now be completed in 10–20 minutes.

Although these new MRI techniques have only recently been introduced clinically, the quantity of relevant data provided by integrated MR exams has already led to speculation that MRI may soon partially replace conventional computed tomography (CT) as the preferred imaging modality in acute stroke. MRI is already on its way to becoming the standard of care in acute stroke in major institutions in both the US and Europe [1]. However, there have also been recent advances in CT technology (in particular CT-angiography, CT-perfusion imaging), which considerably improve the diagnostic yield of CT. Therefore, it can be expected that both advanced MRI and CT techniques will play a major role in the future emergency diagnostic work-up of stroke patients.

Most of the new MR techniques discussed here are already routinely used in clinical practice. There is a general consensus that MRI can increase diagnostic confidence compared to conventional CT in the acute stroke setting, and can lead to a more focused evaluation of the underlying cause of stroke. However, the precise role of the new MR techniques in guiding patient management (e.g., patient selection for thrombolysis) is still under intense investigation.

In this chapter, we will:
- briefly outline the basic technical principles underlying the main new MRI techniques: DWI and PWI. (For a detailed description of technical aspects, the reader is referred to several recent reviews [2–5])
- review current pathophysiologic concepts that are relevant to the interpretation of acute stroke MRI
- outline the role of new MRI techniques in the diagnostic evaluation and management of acute stroke patients

Techniques

The new techniques typically require MRI scanners and gradients that are capable of ultrafast imaging methods, such as echoplanar imaging (EPI). Most of the newer scanners, which typically operate at 1.5 Tesla (T), fulfill these requirements.

DWI

In conventional MRI, signal intensity depends on the density of water protons and various relaxation processes (T1, T2, and T2*). In DWI, additional strong diffusion-sensitizing gradients are used to make the MRI signal sensitive to the random movement of water protons (Brownian motion; see **Figure 1**). In entirely stationary protons, the symmetrical diffusion-sensitizing gradients will lead to a dephasing and then an exact rephasing of the water protons in each voxel (large MRI signal). However, movement of water protons due to diffusion will lead to phase shifts and subsequently imperfect rephasing, which in turn leads to a smaller DWI signal [4]. Therefore, areas of reduced diffusion appear bright on DWI images.

Until a few years ago, the greatest problem with DWI in the acute setting was macroscopic patient motion. However, with new EPI sequences, which can produce image slices in a single shot in ~50–100 ms, patient motion is no longer a problem. With these ultrafast sequences, 20–30 slices covering the whole brain can be obtained in just a few seconds. In fact, DWI is now substantially more robust against gross patient motion than all conventional MRI techniques and excellent quality DWI can be obtained even in critically ill patients. One drawback to using DWI with single-shot EPI is that distortions are frequently found at the base of the skull due to the large susceptibility changes between air, bone, and brain. This is hardly ever a diagnostic problem, but it can influence the measurement of lesion volumes.

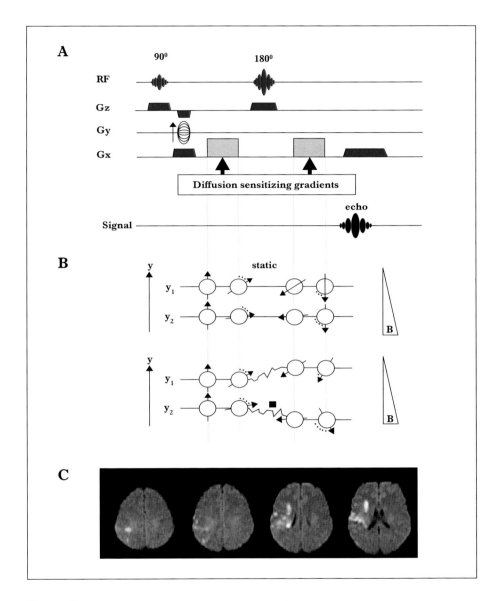

Figure 1. Diffusion-weighted imaging – technical aspects.
In A, a typical pulse-sequence is shown with two strong diffusion-sensitizing gradients (red) arranged symmetrically around the 180° radiofrequency (RF) pulse. The first of the two diffusion-sensitizing gradients leads to a dephasing of water protons, while the second gradient leads to an exact rephasing, provided the water protons do not move between the gradients. If the water protons change their location between the two gradients, as in diffusion, the second gradient will lead to an incorrect rephasing (B). Therefore, the spins will not perfectly realign after the second gradient, which results in a smaller signal. Conversely, if diffusion is restricted, the spins will rephase more accurately, leading to a stronger signal on the diffusion weighted images (such as in the case shown in C, where multiple areas of diffusion-weighted imaging (DWI) hyperintensity can be found in the right middle cerebral artery territory).

PWI

PWI can be performed by using either bolus-tracking (BT-PWI) (see **Figure 2A**) or arterial spin labeling (ASL) techniques [6]. In the acute stroke setting, only BT-PWI techniques are used due to the relatively long examination time and theoretical problems with long transit times in ASL techniques. In a typical BT-PWI exam, multislice T2*-weighted images are acquired every 1–2 seconds for 1–2 minutes. Some groups use serial T1- or T2-weighted images for PWI calculations, but these methods are less common [7]. The number of slices that can be scanned, and thus the coverage, depends on the speed of the system. On most modern scanners, 10–20 slices can be obtained, preferably with the same angulation as the DWI scans. The exogenous contrast agent (e.g., gadolinium diethylene-triamine penta-acetic acid [DTPA]) is injected into the antecubital vein as a bolus, typically with the use of a power injector (typical flow rate: 5 mL/s). When the contrast agent reaches the brain, the MRI signal drops and then recovers again as the contrast agent is washed out (see **Figure 2B**).

Following acquisition of the PWI raw data, the images need to be postprocessed. On some of the newer systems this is done automatically. Typically, various hemodynamic parameters are calculated from the signal-time curve in each pixel (see **Figure 2C**). The most commonly calculated parameters are time-to-peak (TTP), mean transit time (MTT), relative cerebral blood flow (rCBF), and volume (rCBV). The advantages of TTP maps are that they are very sensitive as well as easy to calculate and interpret, since they simply display the time between the beginning of the exam and the maximal signal drop in each pixel. Areas with reduced perfusion are identified as areas with delays in TTP. The other maps, although more difficult to calculate, have the advantage that they are physiologically more meaningful than the TTP maps. Various methods have been developed to calculate absolute flow values, all relying on the determination of an arterial input function and subsequent deconvolution methods. However, in acute stroke patients these methods have not yet been validated, and both bolus delays and bolus dispersion due to large vessel occlusion can probably lead to substantial errors. Therefore, at the present time, PWI should still be regarded as a technique yielding relative values in patients with acute stroke.

Other MRI techniques

Other promising new MRI techniques include contrast-enhanced MRA (CE-MRA), rapid spectroscopic imaging techniques, and diffusion tensor imaging. With CE-MRA, it may become possible to reduce the time currently required for the standard time-of-flight technique (~3 minutes), which would be particularly important in very ill patients. The technique has already been used successfully for the extracranial circulation [8], but experience with the

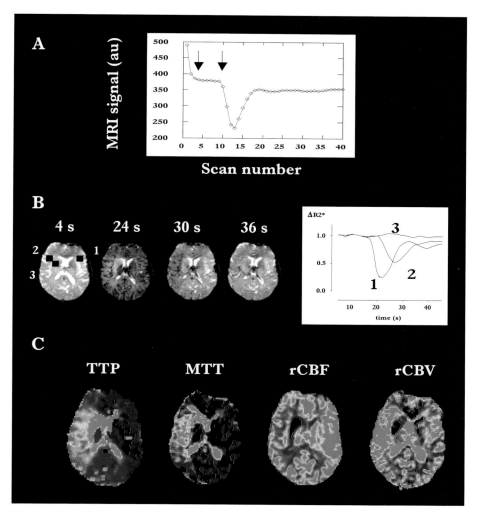

Figure 2 A–C. Perfusion-weighted imaging.
In acute stroke, perfusion-weighted imaging (PWI) is routinely performed as a bolus-tracking technique, where a contrast agent is injected intravenously (first arrow in **A**) during the acquisition of serial T2*-weighted images. When the contrast agent arrives in the brain (second arrow in **A**), the magnetic resonance imaging (MRI) signal decreases transiently. In the example shown in **B**, 40 T2*-weighted images were acquired every 2 seconds (only four selected images are shown). In normal tissue (1) the signal decrease is more pronounced than in the ischemic cortex (2), while in the ischemic core no signal drop is detectable (3). From the raw data, several parameter maps (**C**) can be calculated on a pixel-by-pixel basis. Commonly generated maps include time-to-peak, mean transit time, relative cerebral blood flow and volume maps (TTP, MTT, rCBF, rCBV) (modified with permission from [5]).

intracranial circulation is still limited. With rapid spectroscopic imaging techniques, determination of lactate (and *N*-acetyl aspartate [NAA]) levels in critically affected regions could lead to improvements in predicting tissue outcome [9]. In contrast, diffusion tensor imaging [10] has the potential to become an important tool in the subacute phase for the tracking of residual fiber connectivity, and may be particularly interesting when used in combination with functional MRI (fMRI). However, none of these newer techniques have assumed a definitive role in the acute setting.

Data processing

The ongoing development of faster data processing techniques, which will drastically reduce the total time required for a complete integrated MR examination, is equally important as the development of new imaging techniques. On some of the newer scanners, complete examinations with DWI, PWI, MRA, T2*-weighted imaging, and several conventional sequences can be completed in less than 10 minutes.

Pathophysiologic insights from DWI and PWI

Basic mechanisms

In both experimental and human stroke, severely ischemic tissue becomes hyperintense on DWI within minutes after symptom onset, indicating restricted diffusion of water protons [11,12]. The degree of diffusion restriction can be quantified by a parameter known as the 'apparent diffusion coefficient' (ADC), which typically drops to <80% of control levels in severely affected tissue.

From a pathophysiologic perspective, the ADC decline during ischemia is believed to be due to cytotoxic edema caused by cellular energy failure in the ischemic region (for a detailed discussion of the potential mechanisms involved, see [2,13]). Total depletion of high-energy phosphates (e.g., adenosine triphosphate [ATP]) leads to ion-pump failure, which in turn results in a shift of water from the extracellular space to the intracellular environment, where diffusion is more restricted. In addition, the reduction of the extracellular space leads to a diffusion restriction for the remaining extracellular water molecules (see **Figure 3**). Mild cytotoxic edema associated with increases in lactate and tissue pH, but without (complete) depletion of ATP, can also lead to a decline in ADC values, but probably not to values below ~80% of preischemic values. The exact biophysical factors contributing to the apparent diffusion restriction are still under debate. However, it is generally accepted that cytotoxic edema plays a major role in this process. Therefore, DWI is a technique that primarily detects *metabolic* disturbances of ischemic tissue rather than perfusion abnormalities.

There is general agreement that the decrease in rCBF needs to be relatively severe for DWI to become positive. In humans, no *absolute* flow thresholds have been

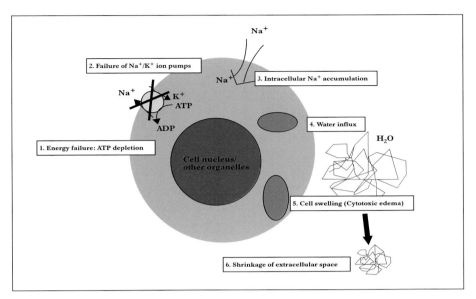

Figure 3. Diffusion-weighted imaging – pathophysiology.
Schematic diagram depicting the cascade of events leading to restricted diffusion in cerebral ischemia. Energy failure with subsequent depletion of adenosine triphosphate (ATP) is believed to be the initial event leading to cytotoxic edema. Cytotoxic edema is associated with restricted diffusion of water molecules, due to the shift of extracellular water into the intracellular space as well as the reduction of the extracellular space.

established. With PWI, rCBF values of ~40% (of contralateral CBF values) have been found at the border of DWI lesions [14,15]. Assuming that average contralateral rCBF values are around 40–50 mL/100 g/min, this would translate into a threshold of 16–20 mL/100 g/min, which is in the 'penumbral range' and slightly above the commonly cited threshold for irreversible tissue injury of ~12 mL/100 g/min [16]. This value correlates with experimental data, where thresholds of 20–41 mL/100 g/min have been found [13]. In rats, an ADC of ≤77% of contralateral values (and rCBF ≤18 mL/100 g/min) was found in regions with depleted ATP [17], indicating that ADC values of less than ~80% are associated with ischemia sufficiently severe to cause total depletion of ATP [18].

However, there are several problems with the determination of flow thresholds for DWI. First, it should be noted that the accuracy of rCBF values measured with PWI is relatively poor. Secondly, systematic clinical studies correlating DWI with other, more established methods for the measurement of rCBF (e.g., positron emission tomography [PET]) have not been reported. Finally, flow thresholds for DWI are probably not static, but change with time; as shown in animal studies, the rCBF threshold shifts to higher values as time from ischemia onset increases [18].

In summary, DWI appears to be a highly reliable indicator of critical ischemia, but there appears to be no single flow threshold.

Are DWI lesions reversible?

In the clinical setting, acute DWI lesions invariably evolve into areas of infarction, with few exceptions reported in the literature [19–21], which leads to the assumption that areas of hyperintensity on DWI indicate irreversible tissue injury.

This view has recently been challenged by Kidwell et al. [22], who found that early DWI lesions were partially reversible after intra-arterial thrombolysis. This indicates that DWI abnormalities may be partially reversed if reperfusion is achieved rapidly. Their data are consistent with the experimental situation, where – particularly in the periphery of DWI lesions – rCBF is initially often above the threshold for irreversible tissue injury and ATP depletion may be incomplete [17].

However, when considering the potential reversibility of DWI lesions, it has to be kept in mind that the ADC reversal in the early reperfusion phase may only be transient, at least in experimental models. Particularly after short periods of ischemia, a secondary ADC decline can occur several hours later [23,24]. Therefore, to accurately assess the outcome of the initially DWI-positive regions, final infarct size must be determined sufficiently late (after several days). The mechanisms underlying the transient ADC reversal have not been determined in detail, but are likely to include both true transient metabolic tissue recovery, as well as processes that make DWI relatively insensitive to ischemic tissue injury in the early reperfusion phase.

In summary, both clinical and experimental data show that hyperintense regions on DWI do not necessarily indicate irreversible tissue injury, but the probability of tissue recovery is generally very low. The most salvageable hyperintense regions on DWI exist in the periphery of the lesions in the hyperacute phase if reperfusion is achieved rapidly.

The DWI–PWI mismatch

One of the exciting aspects of the new MRI techniques is that they allow, at least to a certain extent, the identification of viable 'tissue at risk'. In the first hours after symptom onset, perfusion abnormalities on PWI are typically larger than the corresponding DWI lesions ('DWI–PWI mismatch': see **Figure 4**), but the DWI lesions often grow into the mismatch region over time (see **Figures 5** and **6**) [25–27]. Therefore, the DWI–PWI mismatch region is believed to represent potentially salvageable tissue at risk of infarction [14]. In addition, as outlined above, the periphery of the DWI lesion may also include viable tissue.

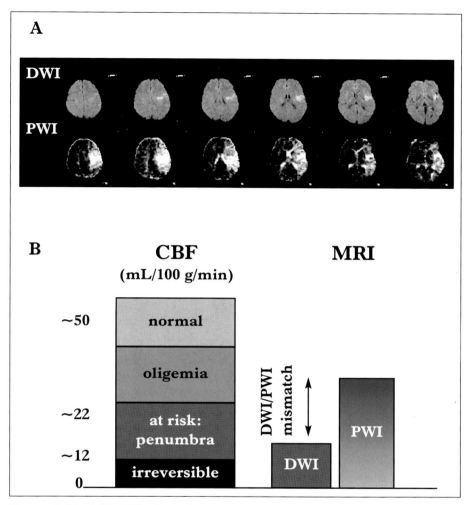

Figure 4. The DWI–PWI mismatch.
An example of a large diffusion-weighted imaging–perfusion-weighted imaging (DWI–PWI) mismatch (perfusion deficit larger than the diffusion lesion) is shown in A. This pattern is frequently found in the first few hours after stroke onset, as shown in this patient, and indicates the presence of still salvageable tissue at risk. The schematic in B shows a (partially speculative) comparison of flow thresholds for DWI and PWI, and tissue viability. From this schematic it is evident that there is a substantial overlap between the true 'penumbra' and the DWI–PWI mismatch, but the thresholds are not identical.
CBF: cerebral blood flow; MRI: magnetic resonance imaging.

However, the final outcome of the DWI–PWI mismatch region has remained relatively unpredictable in individual patients. This is partially due to the fact that reperfusion may occur at unpredictable time points following the acute MRI study (see **Figure 5**). In addition, it is clear that not all of the DWI–PWI mismatch will be at equal risk of infarction, but differentiating between critical ischemia and oligemia is still difficult with PWI. The magnitude of the TTP-delay is a helpful

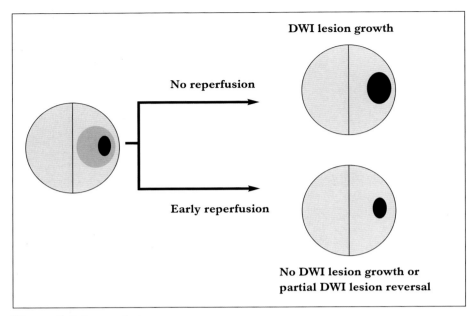

Figure 5. Infarct evolution.
Schematic showing diffusion-weighted imaging (DWI) lesion evolution depending on the time of reperfusion.

parameter in this respect, with delays of at least 4–6 seconds (compared to the contralateral side) indicating critical ischemia (see **Figure 6**) [28]. However, there is no broad consensus as to which perfusion parameters (TTP, MTT, rCBF, rCBV) are optimal for the calculation of the mismatch and the prediction of tissue outcome. In patients with proximal carotid artery stenosis or occlusion, the region at risk may be substantially overestimated as these patients frequently have pre-existing large perfusion abnormalities due to the hemodynamic effect of the carotid disease [15]; in these patients, only relatively small subregions of the large perfusion deficits may become critically ischemic at the time of stroke onset due to distal embolization.

One of the most important independent parameters predicting DWI lesion expansion (into the mismatch region) is absent middle cerebral artery (MCA) flow on MRA. Rordorf et al. found a far greater increase in DWI lesion size in patients with MCA main stem occlusion than in patients with branch occlusions [29]. In addition, Barber et al. found that MCA occlusion on MRA is predictive of the presence of 'penumbral patterns' (essentially a positive DWI–PWI mismatch) with a greater increase in DWI lesion size than in patients without MCA occlusion [30].

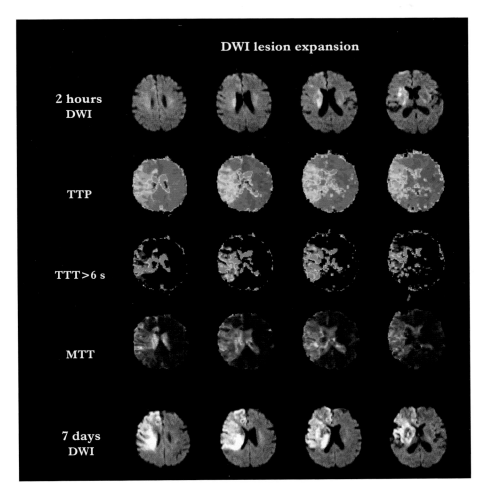

Figure 6. DWI lesion expansion.
In this patient presenting 2 hours after stroke onset, the diffusion-weighted imaging (DWI) lesion expanded dramatically between the acute and the follow-up scan at 7 days. Dramatic DWI lesion expansion is most commonly found in patients with occlusions of the M1-segment of the middle cerebral artery or T-occlusions of the internal carotid artery, both of which are typically associated with extensive perfusion abnormalities (acquired in collaboration with the Departments of Neurology and Radiology, Düsseldorf, Germany).
MTT: mean transit time; TTP: time-to-peak; TTT: time-to-treat.

Clinical applications

Identification of the clinically relevant lesion and classification of stroke subtype

In the majority of acute stroke patients, DWI alone will reveal at least one lesion, even in the first hours after symptom onset. Acute lesions are hyperintense on DWI (with correspondingly low ADC values), and can be identified as the clinically relevant lesion [31]. This is in contrast to older lesions, which have a (pseudo-) normal or abnormally high ADC. In human stroke, the ADC typically remains low for several days to weeks, and then increases [32]. Rapid identification of the clinically relevant lesion has made DWI the centerpiece of MRI studies for acute stroke. Nevertheless, a complete assessment of the ischemic tissue including the identification of viable tissue at risk is only possible with a combination of DWI with PWI, MRA, and conventional MRI.

Occasionally, DWI will be negative in the acute setting despite the clinical suspicion of stroke. In about half of these patients, ischemic infarcts will be found at follow-up [33]. In these cases, PWI is an essential component of the acute MRI examination, since many of these patients will have substantial PWI deficits. This constellation (PWI, but no DWI abnormality) probably indicates that the ischemic tissue is still potentially salvageable at the time of the acute scan. If the initial PWI exam is normal as well, ischemic disease is still not entirely ruled out, since lacunar stroke, especially if located in the brain stem, may occasionally escape detection by DWI and PWI [34]. In addition, patients with transient ischemic attacks can have entirely negative DWI and PWI studies [21], but probably only in the phase when their symptoms are either rapidly resolving or already absent again. However, in our experience, completely negative DWI and PWI studies are very rare in ischemic disease with persisting symptoms, and the search for nonischemic causes (e.g., focal epilepsy, migraine, unmasking of prior neurological deficits by intercurrent illness) should be intensified.

A major advantage of integrated MRI exams is that they considerably increase the diagnostic confidence in the acute setting and allow a highly accurate diagnosis of stroke subtype. This, in turn, can have a substantial impact on the diagnostic evaluation of the patient regarding the underlying cause of stroke and may alter patient management [35]. Typical examples include: single small subcortical DWI lesions suggestive of small vessel disease [36], where a limited neurodiagnostic evaluation may be sufficient; and either single large or multiple small cortical and subcortical DWI lesions suggesting cerebral embolization [37], where a proximal source of embolization should be searched for carefully (e.g., cardiac disease including a patent foramen ovale, aortic arch atherosclerosis, or carotid disease).

Patient selection for thrombolysis

The new MRI techniques have the potential to become very useful tools in the triage of acute stroke patients for thrombolysis with tissue plasminogen activator (tPA), which has become the standard treatment for selected patients within the first 3 hours after symptom onset [38,39]. Currently, CT is still used in most centers prior to thrombolytic therapy to exclude intracerebral hemorrhage (ICH). In addition, conventional CT may show early infarct signs such as parenchymal hypointensity or sulcal effacement [40], but these signs are often subtle, if present at all. In contrast, the new MRI techniques can provide a more complete assessment of the extent and severity of ischemic tissue injury, and the images are easier to interpret than CT scans. However, as with CT, little specific information is available on how best to select patients for intravenous thrombolysis in the 0–3-hour time window based on their acute MRI. In the following text, we summarize factors that may form a rational basis for treatment decisions (although they have not been proven to improve outcome in systematic studies).

From a theoretical point of view, patients with little irreversible ischemic tissue damage, but large areas of tissue at risk due to large vessel occlusion, should be ideal candidates for treatment with tPA. As a first approximation, this translates into patients with a small DWI lesion, a large DWI–PWI mismatch, and absent MCA flow on MRA. This is also the group of patients in whom the most pronounced increase in DWI lesion size may be expected after the acute scan (see **Figure 6**) [29]. Conversely, early reperfusion has been found to be associated with significantly smaller final infarct size and a better neurologic outcome in these patients, indicating that DWI lesion expansion may be potentially prevented and that this is clinically relevant [41–43]. However, although early reperfusion appears to be highly beneficial, it has not been proven that tPA treatment is more beneficial in this subgroup than in other patient subgroups. While tPA treatment has been shown to increase the likelihood of reperfusion, it is unclear how frequently reperfusion will occur early enough to prevent DWI lesion expansion.

Various other patient subgroups are unlikely to benefit from thrombolysis. Clearly, patients with a perfusion deficit that is already smaller than the DWI lesion due to spontaneous clot lysis are unlikely to benefit from treatment. The outcome of thrombolysis in patients with a DWI lesion that is similar in size to the PWI deficit is not known. Since early DWI lesions can resolve (at least partially) after intra-arterial thrombolysis [22], it may be argued that these patients could also benefit. However, this may be the case in only a small subgroup of patients with this DWI–PWI pattern, and differentiating these patients from those without residual tissue at risk is not yet possible. Similarly, the utility of thrombolysis in patients with lacunar stroke due to small vessel disease, who typically have a favorable outcome even without treatment, has not been resolved. In the National Institute of Neurological Disorders and Stroke (NINDS) tPA trial, patients with a lacunar syndrome also benefited from treatment [44], but the mechanisms underlying this treatment effect are unclear. In addition, lacunar stroke was only defined clinically in the NINDS tPA trial, which makes interpretation of this finding difficult; future trials will have to determine whether or not patients with lacunar stroke defined by imaging criteria will benefit from thrombolysis.

Thrombolytic therapy in the 3–6-hour time window

Currently, no data exist showing a benefit of intravenous tPA treatment in the 3–6-hour time window [45], although there is general agreement that some patients can benefit even after the first 3 hours. Randomized trials are underway investigating whether MRI can be used to select those patients who will benefit from intravenous thrombolysis in the 3–6-hour time frame [46], but no results are available. However, the PROACT II trial studying intra-arterial thrombolysis with pro-urokinase [47] found a significant benefit for patients with MCA main stem occlusion presenting in the 3–6-hour time window. For this reason, intra-arterial thrombolysis is currently preferred in the 3–6-hour time window in most specialized centers.

From a practical point of view, MRI is undoubtedly helpful in the selection of patients for intra-arterial thrombolysis [48]. Most importantly, MRA may be highly suggestive of MCA occlusion, making these patients ideal candidates for angiography and intra-arterial thrombolysis. Conversely, conventional angiography will be unnecessary in patients with a normal flow signal over the MCA. In addition, the aggressiveness of the therapeutic approach will be influenced by the DWI–PWI pattern. If there is a relatively small DWI lesion, the benefit can be expected to be great. On the other hand, if there is a dense DWI lesion affecting most of the MCA territory, the potential benefit of thrombolytic therapy is probably small.

The situation is currently unclear in patients with presumed distal internal carotid artery (ICA) occlusion ('T-occlusion'). Our approach is to attempt intra-arterial thrombolysis in these patients, but reperfusion is probably achieved less frequently than in MCA occlusion. Moreover, localization of the precise site of occlusion may be difficult with MRA alone, since both proximal and distal ICA occlusion may lead to minimal or absent flow in the distal ICA, or may coexist. This is a practical and as yet unresolved problem, since it may be difficult or even impossible to pass (or bypass) the proximal occlusion site during angiography to reach the (more important) distal embolus.

Detection of hyperacute hemorrhage

Hyperacute hemorrhage may be difficult to detect with conventional MRI in the first 6 hours after symptom onset. This has led to widespread skepticism about the capability of MRI to detect acute hemorrhage. However, recent studies have convincingly shown that susceptibility- or T2*-weighted gradient echo MR

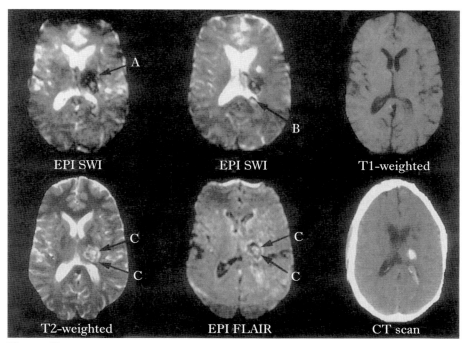

Figure 7. MRI of hyperacute hemorrhage.
T2*-weighted images, or susceptibility-weighted images (SWI), are now routinely obtained in acute stroke examinations due to the unique sensitivity of these sequences for the detection of acute parenchymal hemorrhage. In the example shown here, echoplanar imaging (EPI)-SWI was obtained 79 minutes after sudden onset of right-sided weakness and numbness. The two contiguous slices on SWI show signal loss in the left thalamus (arrow A) with extension in the posterior limb of the internal capsule and invasion of the posterior horn of the left lateral ventricle (arrow B). T2*-weighted imaging and fluid-attenuated inversion recovery (FLAIR) show the same lesion present on SWI as an area of increased signal intensity with a periphery of signal loss (arrow C) and a surrounding rim of increased signal intensity, most likely due to vasogenic edema (reproduced with permission from [50]).

sequences ('bleed screen') are highly sensitive for the detection of intraparenchymal hemorrhage (see **Figure 7**) [49–51]. The area of hemorrhage is usually easy to identify on these images as a region of decreased signal intensity or with a mixed hyperintense/hypointense pattern.

Due to the promising results of these preliminary reports [49–51], some centers with extensive experience in acute stroke MRI have now started to use MRI as the sole imaging modality before thrombolysis. However, in all cases of doubt an additional CT is still recommended until larger randomized studies have been published reporting a similar sensitivity and specificity of T2*-weighted MRI compared to CT for the detection of intraparenchymal hemorrhage.

It is yet to be decided whether or not patients with very small hemorrhages (so called 'microbleeds') on T2*-weighted scans should be excluded from treatment with tPA. These microbleeds are relatively common [52], particularly in patients with microangiopathy, and are typically only seen on MRI (not on CT). There is convincing evidence that patients with microbleeds are at an increased risk of spontaneous or warfarin-associated hemorrhage, but it is unclear whether they are also at an increased risk of symptomatic hemorrhagic transformation following treatment with thrombolytics.

Finally, it should be noted that the exclusion of subarachnoid hemorrhage (SAH) with MRI is not yet possible. Unfortunately, the T2*-weighted EPI-sequences, which are the most sensitive for the detection of blood in the acute setting, suffer from relatively severe susceptibility artifacts at the base of the skull, where the blood typically accumulates in SAH. Recent studies have reported other sequences, e.g., fluid attenuated inversion recovery (FLAIR)- and proton-density weighted sequences, with a high sensitivity for the detection of acute SAH [53,54]. However, until further studies show a similar sensitivity compared to CT, MRI is not yet recommended in cases of suspected SAH.

Other emerging applications

A number of recent intriguing reports indicate that the new MRI techniques may also become useful in other areas of stroke management including the following:

- prediction of hemorrhagic transformation (HT) following tPA treatment of ischemic stroke. Tong et al. showed that patients with areas of very low ADC in the ischemic area are at increased risk of secondary HT [55]. Areas of very low ADC may indicate particularly severe ischemia leading to early blood–brain barrier damage, which is believed to be associated with an increased risk of HT. Identification of those patients at an increased risk of symptomatic HT and exclusion of those patients from tPA treatment may ultimately increase overall patient benefit from thrombolysis

- prediction of malignant MCA infarction. Oppenheim et al. recently reported that patients with a large DWI lesion volume (>145 cm^3) frequently develop malignant MCA infarction with massive edema, typically requiring decompressive surgery as a life-saving measure [56]. Since early surgery in these patients has been shown to result in an improved outcome, reliable early predictors of subsequent malignant MCA infarction would be very valuable

- posterior circulation ischemia. Particularly in basilar artery thrombosis, which is associated with a very high mortality, the possibility to identify basilar artery occlusion with MRA as well as the extent of severe ischemic tissue damage in critical brain regions (i.e., the brain stem) with DWI may become useful in the triage of patients for intra-arterial thrombolysis in the future [57]

Conclusion

Over the last 10 years, MRI has evolved into a very valuable tool for the evaluation of acute stroke patients. The development of advanced MRI techniques such as DWI, PWI, and high-speed MRA has revolutionized our ability to investigate ischemic pathophysiology in individual patients. Due to the greater quantity of relevant data provided for MRI compared to conventional CT, many centers have now started to use these techniques routinely.

At present, the precise role of the new MRI methods in the selection of acute stroke patients for various therapies is still under intense investigation. However, we anticipate that treatment stratification in the acute stroke setting will soon be possible on the basis of individual MRI patterns.

References

1. Hacke W, Warach S. Diffusion-weighted MRI as an evolving standard of care in acute stroke. *Neurology* 2000;54:1548–9.
2. Baird AE, Warach S. Magnetic resonance imaging of acute stroke. *J Cereb Blood Flow Metab* 1998;18:583–609.
3. Beauchamp NJ, Jr., Barker PB, Wang PY et al. Imaging of acute cerebral ischemia. *Radiology* 1999;212:307–24.
4. Moseley ME, Butts K. Diffusion and Perfusion. In: Stark D, Bradley WG, editors. *Magnetic Resonance Imaging*. 3rd ed. St. Louis: Mosby, 1999:1515–38.
5. Neumann-Haefelin T, Moseley ME, Albers GW. New magnetic resonance imaging methods for cerebrovascular disease: emerging clinical applications. *Ann Neurol* 2000;47:559–70.
6. Calamante F, Thomas DL, Pell GS et al. Measuring cerebral blood flow using magnetic resonance imaging techniques. *J Cereb Blood Flow Metab* 1999;19:701–35.
7. Moody AR, Martel A, Kenton A et al. Contrast-reduced imaging of tissue concentration and arterial level (CRITICAL) for assessment of cerebral hemodynamics in acute stroke by magnetic resonance. *Invest Radiol* 2000;35:401–11.
8. Remonda L, Heid O, Schroth G. Carotid artery stenosis, occlusion, and pseudo-occlusion: first-pass, gadolinium-enhanced, three-dimensional MR angiography—preliminary study. *Radiology* 1998;209:95–102.
9. Franke C, Brinker G, Pillekamp F et al. Probability of metabolic tissue recovery after thrombolytic treatment of experimental stroke: a magnetic resonance spectroscopic imaging study in rat brain. *J Cereb Blood Flow Metab* 2000;20:583–91.
10. Basser PJ, Pajevic S, Pierpaoli C et al. In vivo fiber tractography using DT-MRI data. *Magn Reson Med* 2000;44:625–32.
11. Moseley ME, Cohen Y, Mintorovitch J et al. Early detection of regional cerebral ischemia in cats: comparison of diffusion- and T2-weighted MRI and spectroscopy. *Magn Reson Med* 1990;14:330–46.
12. Warach S, Chien D, Li W et al. Fast magnetic resonance diffusion-weighted imaging of acute human stroke. *Neurology* 1992;42:1717–23.
13. Hossmann K–A, Hoehn-Berlage M. Diffusion and perfusion MR imaging of cerebral ischemia. *Cerebrovasc Brain Metab Rev* 1995;7:187–217.
14. Schlaug G, Benfield A, Baird AE et al. The ischemic penumbra: operationally defined by diffusion and perfusion MRI. *Neurology* 1999;53:1528–37.
15. Neumann-Haefelin T, Wittsack HJ, Fink GR et al. Diffusion- and perfusion-weighted MRI: influence of severe carotid artery stenosis on the DWI/PWI mismatch in acute stroke. *Stroke* 2000;31:1311–7.

16. Heiss WD. Ischemic penumbra: evidence from functional imaging in man. *J Cereb Blood Flow Metab* 2000;20:1276–93.

17. Hoehn–Berlage M, Norris DG, Kohno K et al. Evolution of regional changes in apparent diffusion coefficient during focal ischemia of rat brain: the relationship of quantitative diffusion NMR imaging to reduction in cerebral blood flow and metabolic disturbances. *J Cereb Blood Flow Metab* 1995;15:1002–11.

18. Kohno K, Hoehn–Berlage M, Mies G et al. Relationship between diffusion-weighted MR images, cerebral blood flow, and energy state in experimental brain infarction. *Magn Reson Imaging* 1995;13:73–80.

19. Marks MP, de Crespigny A, Lentz D et al. Acute and chronic stroke: navigated spin-echo diffusion-weighted MR imaging. *Radiology* 1996;199:403–8.

20. Lecouvet FE, Duprez TP, Raymackers JM et al. Resolution of early diffusion-weighted and FLAIR MRI abnormalities in a patient with TIA. *Neurology* 1999;52:1085–7.

21. Kidwell CS, Alger JR, Di Salle F et al. Diffusion MRI in patients with transient ischemic attacks. *Stroke* 1999;30:1174–80.

22. Kidwell CS, Saver JL, Mattiello J et al. Thrombolytic reversal of acute human cerebral ischemic injury shown by diffusion/perfusion magnetic resonance imaging. *Ann Neurol* 2000;47:462–9.

23. Li F, Silva MD, Sotak CH et al. Temporal evolution of ischemic injury evaluated with diffusion-, perfusion-, and T2-weighted MRI. *Neurology* 2000;54:689–96.

24. Neumann-Haefelin T, Kastrup A, de Crespigny A et al. Serial MRI after transient focal cerebral ischemia in rats: dynamics of tissue injury, blood-brain barrier damage, and edema formation. *Stroke* 2000;31:1965–73.

25. Baird AE, Benfield A, Schlaug G et al. Enlargement of human cerebral ischemic lesion volumes measured by diffusion-weighted magnetic resonance imaging. *Ann Neurol* 1997;41:581–9.

26. Tong DC, Yenari MA, Albers GW et al. Correlation of perfusion- and diffusion-weighted MRI with NIHSS score in acute (<6.5 hour) ischemic stroke. *Neurology* 1998;50:864–70.

27. Barber PA, Darby DG, Desmond PM et al. Prediction of stroke outcome with echoplanar perfusion- and diffusion- weighted MRI. *Neurology* 1998;51:418–26.

28. Neumann-Haefelin T, Wittsack HJ, Wenserski F et al. Diffusion- and perfusion-weighted MRI: the DWI/PWI mismatch region in acute stroke. *Stroke* 1999;30:159–7.

29. Rordorf G, Koroshetz WJ, Copen WA et al. Regional ischemia and ischemic injury in patients with acute middle cerebral artery stroke as defined by early diffusion-weighted and perfusion-weighted MRI. *Stroke* 1998;29:939–43.

30. Barber PA, Davis SM, Darby DG et al. Absent middle cerebral artery flow predicts the presence and evolution of the ischemic penumbra. *Neurology* 1999;52:1125–32.

31. Lutsep HL, Albers GW, de Crespigny A et al. Clinical utility of diffusion-weighted magnetic resonance imaging in the assessment of ischemic stroke. *Ann Neurol* 1997;41:574–80.

32. Schlaug G, Siewert B, Benfield A et al. Time course of the apparent diffusion coefficient (ADC) abnormality in human stroke. *Neurology* 1997;49:113–9.

33. Ay H, Buonanno FS, Rordorf G et al. Normal diffusion-weighted MRI during stroke-like deficits. *Neurology* 1999;52:1784–92.

34. Oppenheim C, Stanescu R, Dormont D et al. False-negative diffusion-weighted MR findings in acute ischemic stroke. *AJNR Am J Neuroradiol* 2000;21:1434–40.

35. Albers GW, Lansberg MG, Norbash AM et al. Yield of diffusion-weighted MRI for detection of potentially relevant findings in stroke patients. *Neurology* 2000;54:1562–7.

36. Schonewille WJ, Tuhrim S, Singer MB et al. Diffusion-weighted MRI in acute lacunar syndromes: a clinical-radiological correlation study. *Stroke* 1999;30:2066–9.

37. Baird AE, Lovblad KO, Schlaug G et al. Multiple acute stroke syndrome: marker of embolic disease? *Neurology* 2000;54:674–8.

38. The National Institute of Neurological Disorders and Stroke rt-PA Stroke Study Group. Tissue plasminogen activator for acute ischemic stroke. *N Engl J Med* 1995;333:1581–7.

39. Hacke W, Kaste M, Fieschi C et al. Intravenous thrombolysis with recombinant tissue plasminogen activator for acute hemispheric stroke. The European Cooperative Acute Stroke Study (ECASS). *JAMA* 1995;274:1017–25.

40. von Kummer R, Allen KL, Holle R et al. Acute stroke: usefulness of early CT findings before thrombolytic therapy. *Radiology* 1997;205:327–33.

41. Jansen O, Schellinger P, Fiebach J et al. Early recanalisation in acute ischaemic stroke saves tissue at risk defined by MRI. *Lancet* 1999;353:2036–7.

42. Beaulieu C, de Crespigny A, Tong DC et al. Longitudinal magnetic resonance imaging study of perfusion and diffusion in stroke: evolution of lesion volume and correlation with clinical outcome. *Ann Neurol* 1999;46:568–78.

43. Schellinger PD, Jansen O, Fiebach JB et al. Monitoring intravenous recombinant tissue plasminogen activator thrombolysis for acute ischemic stroke with diffusion and perfusion MRI. *Stroke* 2000;31:1318–28.

44. Generalized efficacy of t-PA for acute stroke. Subgroup analysis of the NINDS t-PA Stroke Trial. *Stroke* 1997;28:2119–25.

45. Clark WM, Wissman S, Albers GW et al. Recombinant tissue-type plasminogen activator (Alteplase) for ischemic stroke 3 to 5 hours after symptom onset. The ATLANTIS Study: a randomized controlled trial. Alteplase Thrombolysis for Acute Noninterventional Therapy in Ischemic Stroke. *JAMA* 1999;282:2019–26.

46. Albers GW. Expanding the window for thrombolytic therapy in acute stroke: the potential role of acute MRI for patient selection. *Stroke* 1999;30:2230–7.

47. Furlan A, Higashida R, Wechsler L et al. Intra-arterial prourokinase for acute ischemic stroke. The PROACT II study: a randomized controlled trial. Prolyse in Acute Cerebral Thromboembolism. *JAMA* 1999;282:2003–11.

48. Sunshine JL, Tarr RW, Lanzieri CF et al. Hyperacute stroke: ultrafast MR imaging to triage patients prior to therapy. *Radiology* 1999;212:325–32.

49. Patel MR, Edelman RR, Warach S. Detection of hyperacute primary intraparenchymal hemorrhage by magnetic resonance imaging. *Stroke* 1996;27:2321–4.

50. Linfante I, Llinas RH, Caplan LR et al. MRI features of intracerebral hemorrhage within 2 hours from symptom onset. *Stroke* 1999;30:2263–7.

51. Schellinger PD, Jansen O, Fiebach JB et al. A standardized MRI stroke protocol: comparison with CT in hyperacute intracerebral hemorrhage. *Stroke* 1999;30:765–8.

52. Roob G, Fazekas F. Magnetic resonance imaging of cerebral microbleeds. *Curr Opin Neurol* 2000;13:69–73.

53. Singer MB, Atlas SW, Drayer BP. Subarachnoid space disease: diagnosis with fluid-attenuated inversion-recovery MR imaging and comparison with gadolinium-enhanced spin-echo MR imaging–blinded reader study. *Radiology* 1998;208:417–22.

54. Wiesmann M, Mayer TE, Medele R et al. Diagnosis of acute subarachnoid hemorrhage at 1.5 Tesla using proton-density weighted FSE and MRI sequences. *Radiologe* 1999;39:860–5.

55. Tong DC, Adami A, Moseley ME et al. Relationship between apparent diffusion coefficient and subsequent hemorrhagic transformation following acute ischemic stroke. *Stroke* 2000;31:2378–84.

56. Oppenheim C, Samson Y, Manai R et al. Prediction of malignant middle cerebral artery infarction by diffusion-weighted imaging. *Stroke* 2000;31:2175–81.

57. Caplan L. Posterior circulation ischemia: then, now, and tomorrow. The Thomas Willis Lecture-2000. *Stroke* 2000;31:2011–23.

4

CTA and MRA in stroke

Olav Jansen

Introduction

Computed tomography-angiography (CTA) and magnetic resonance angiography (MRA) are two noninvasive techniques that can be used to evaluate the vascular system. While CTA is an x-ray based technique and always requires contrast administration, MRA is more prone to artifacts. However, both techniques can be combined with conventional slice techniques, allowing a multimodal approach to investigation of vascular diseases.

In this chapter, the advantages and disadvantages of CTA and MRA techniques, and their use in different vascular diseases are discussed.

CT-angiography

CTA is a contrast enhanced CT-technique which produces three-dimensional (3-D) images from arterial or venous vessels. Unlike conventional angiography, CTA only provides morphologic data from vessels and no hemodynamic information. However, the source images from this technique incorporate both the vessels and the surrounding tissue.

Techniques

With the introduction of the spiral technique, CT has become an excellent tool to investigate not only the parenchymal tissue and bone, but also arterial and venous vessels. The main advantages of the spiral CT technique are its speed and the volumetric nature of the data it acquires. The spiral technique also opens the possibility for qualitative evaluation of parenchymal perfusion (perfusion CT). According to the generation of the scanner, spiral CT allows data acquisition of the circle of Willis, the vessels of the entire brain or – with the new generation of multislice scanners – evaluation of the arterial vessels from the aortic arch to the vertex.

In order to obtain optimal images of arteries (or veins), opacification of those vessels that are not to be evaluated in the current scan should be minimized. Opacification of vessels is created by intravenous administration of contrast media. The goal is to attain the highest intravascular contrast possible in those vessels which are to be evaluated. Techniques are available to optimize contrast administration and minimize the amount of contrast required. The most efficient method is to predict the time from injection to peak arterial contrast concentration. This is possible using dynamic scans; one location is repeatedly scanned after administration of a test bolus, and a time-density curve is created. This procedure is done once in each patient. State of the art scanners have implied software programs that are able to detect the bolus arrival of the contrast media with an initial dynamic scan and start the subsequent spiral scan automatically. However, especially in emergency situations, most institutions make an approximate calculation of the necessary delay between contrast injection and CTA scan start (see **Table 1**). Depending on the condition of the cardiovascular system of each patient and the region of interest, the delay times are individually corrected.

Region of interest	Circulation time from antecubital vein to region of interest (seconds)
Carotid bifurcation	15
Circle of Willis	18
Cerebral arteries	20
Cerebral veins	25

Table 1. Common blood circulation times in adults with a healthy cardiovascular system for a contrast bolus injected into the antecubital vein.

As with other modalities, only the source images of CTA provide the correct findings. However, for better demonstration and anatomical orientation, 3-D reconstruction techniques may be helpful in selected cases (see **Figure 1**). Some authors have recommended a subtraction technique to eliminate artifacts from the bone. This method requires two identical spiral scans without any movement of the head; therefore, the patient must be kept completely still. Because cranial CTA is mostly used in patients with acute neurological diseases the feasibility of this subtraction technique is limited. Therefore, removing the skull vault from the image dataset by thresholding and electronically cutting is the preferred technique. Evaluation of the source images is recommended to find the exact diagnosis.

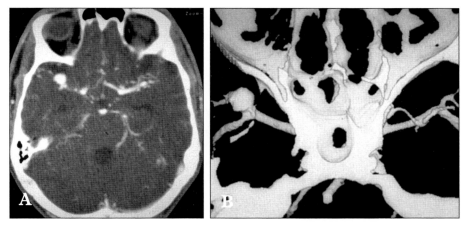

Figure 1. Computed tomography-angiography (CTA) in a patient with aneurysm of the middle cerebral artery bifurcation: source images can demonstrate the aneurysm clearly (A); however, a 3-D angiogram better demonstrates the aneurysm geometry (B).

CTA in brain perfusion

While classical perfusion CT is performed as a dynamic scan on only one location, a spiral CT scan of the entire brain offers information on multiple sites after bolus administration, including:

- the opportunity to evaluate the angiographic situation of the circle of Willis
- visualization of the quality of leptomeningeal collaterals by enhancing the arterial vessels beyond the site of occlusion
- demonstration of an area of minor perfusion by reduced parenchymal enhancement

With an additional subtraction technique, perfused cerebral blood volume (CBV) images can be obtained, which give semiquantitative information about the CBV [1].

CTA in acute arterial ischemic stroke

CTA has shown very high accuracy in determining the competence of the circle of Willis. Wildermuth et al. showed >90% sensitivity and specificity for the diagnosis of vessel occlusion [2]. However, CTA is not as accurate in the evaluation of smaller vessels beyond the MCA bifurcation, and in the quantification of stenoses within the circle of Willis. With the increasing interest in emergency treatment of acute cerebrovascular thrombosis, imaging modalities have become a major part of the pretherapeutic work-up.

While unenhanced CT is able to demonstrate hemorrhagic stroke and early infarct signs with significant prognostic value, CTA is able to show arterial occlusion [3,4]. Furthermore, spiral CTA allows not only the evaluation of the circle of Willis, but also demonstration of brain tissue perfusion. Although this technique results in decreased spatial resolution and lower quality 3-D reconstructed angiograms, it delivers much nonquantitative information about the acute brain perfusion and the integrity of the major brain-supplying arterial vessels. The combined interpretation of results from the spiral CT technique and findings from nonenhanced CT creates a kind of match/mismatch approach between areas with minor perfusion and areas with visible hypodensity (see **Figure 2**). There are no data proving the value of this combined CT diagnostic approach for patients selected before undergoing thrombolytic therapy, however, it may be the best way to provide maximum information with a simple and readily available approach.

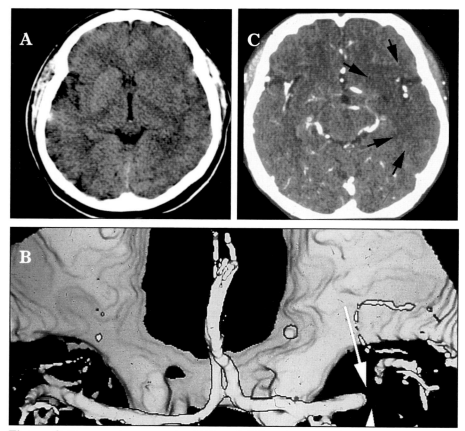

Figure 2. Computed tomography (CT) and CT-angiography (CTA) findings in acute ischemic stroke: unenhanced CT shows early infarct signs in the middle cerebral artery-territory on the left with hypodensity of the lentiform nucleus and obscuration of the insular (A). 3-D reconstruction of CTA-images demonstrate the lateral middle cerebral artery-occlusion (B), while source images of the CTA scan demonstrate an area with minor perfusion and reduced vascular enhancement (C – black arrows).

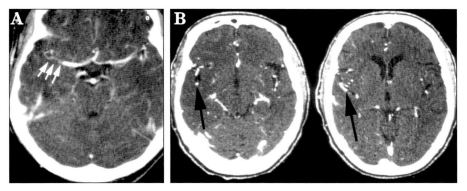

Figure 3. Computed tomography angiography (CTA) in acute right middle cerebral artery (MCA) occlusion with good quality leptomeningeal collaterals: the basal source image shows thrombus in the lateral MCA (A); more cranial images (B) demonstrate retrograde enhancement in slightly dilatated insular branches (black arrows).

In addition, the enhanced spiral scan of the entire brain delivers indirect information about the quality of leptomeningeal collaterals in patients with acute arterial vessel occlusion. The quality of the leptomeningeal collaterals seems to correlate with the grade of enhancement of peripheral branches distal to the occlusion site and the amount of brain tissue with reduced vascular enhancement. It has been demonstrated that the extent of leptomeningeal collaterals as shown by CTA correlated significantly with outcome after intravenous thrombolytic therapy (see **Figure 3**) [2].

CTA is readily available and minimally invasive. It can be performed on all CT scanners with spiral capability and can be performed immediately after standard CT imaging without moving the patient.

Because of the narrow time window for initiation of successful thrombolytic therapy, it is important to note that CTA is a very fast procedure, requiring only an additional 5 minutes examination time in the CT scanner and ~10 minutes reconstruction time. The application of 100 mL nonionic contrast agent for CTA is not a contraindication for subsequent diagnostic or therapeutic digital subtraction angiography (DSA). Idiosyncratic reactions to iodinated contrast agents have been reported, but the use of nonionic agents minimizes the risk of moderate or severe incidents. There is no risk of arterial injury or embolization. CTA can even be applied to severely ill and uncooperative patients due to the speed of imaging. Patients who would have required general anesthesia for DSA have undergone CTA with no sedation or only mild sedation. Contrary to DSA and ultrasound, CTA yields only static images, but hemodynamic or functional information can be inferred by indirect parameters such as visibility of collaterals [1,3].

CTA in carotid dissection

Acute dissection of the internal carotid artery is one of the major causes of arterial ischemic stroke in younger patients. Typical clinical symptoms, such as stroke symptoms combined with neck pain, and specific findings in ultrasound lead to the correct diagnosis in almost all patients. However, because ultrasound is a subjective method with high intermachine and interobserver variability (due to the varying degrees of experience of technicians/doctors observing the results) and because an intimal hematoma can not be verified by ultrasound directly, an objective technique is often required to verify the diagnosis.

In the first 3 days after dissection, the carotid wall hematoma appears hyperdense in CT (see **Figure 4**) and a positive documentation of the lesion is therefore possible with CTA [5,6]. CTA also has a very high accuracy in differentiating total occlusion from pseudo-occlusion in carotid dissection. In clinical experience, this technique is more sensitive than ultrasound, and invasive DSA is not usually required to confirm the diagnosis. CTA can also reveal secondary complications of carotid dissections such as pseudoaneurysm or high-grade stenosis in the infrapetrous part of the internal carotid artery (ICA). During the first 2 days after dissection, direct visualization of the carotid wall hematoma seems to be easier with CT than with MRI because deoxyhemoglobin is hyperdense in CT but hypointense in T1- or T2-weighted MRI. This changes after 3–4 days when deoxyhemoglobin converts to methemoglobin: the hematoma becomes hyperintense and is visible in all MRI sequences.

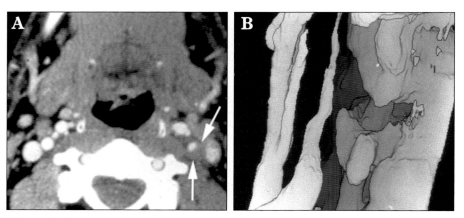

Figure 4. Computed tomography angiography (CTA) in acute dissection of left internal carotid artery: source images show hyperdense hematoma in the carotid wall (white arrows) (A). 3-D angiogram demonstrates the classical tapered sign (B).

CTA in carotid stenosis

The precise degree of carotid artery stenosis and some aspects of plaque morphology are associated with differences in stroke risk and natural history, as well as response to surgery, and may have important management implications, such as the relative appropriateness of surgery. Therefore, precise and objective evaluation of carotid bifurcation disease is strongly recommended. While DSA is still the gold standard in determining the grade of stenosis, ultrasound is widely accepted as an alternative technique in many sites. However, in selected cases, e.g., multiple stenoses, a second imaging modality is required to verify the ultrasound diagnosis.

In a number of recent studies, CTA was compared to DSA and ultrasound in detection and quantification of carotid stenosis [5,7,8]. CTA was found to be a good test for detection of carotid occlusion and for stenoses of >50%. Although the 3-D CTA images are more visually appealing and provide an indication of the location and length of the carotid plaque and the location and orientation of calcifications, they are less reliable in stenosis calculation. For more dependable calculations of stenosis, axial source images have been shown to be the most accurate CTA images and are more precise than maximal intensity projection (MIP) or shaded-surface display (SSD) images [7,9].

However, CTA appears to be less accurate than DSA in describing the grade of stenosis. For CTA the detection rate for 70%–99% stenosis is reported with sensitivity between 67% and 80% in different studies. As this may lead to incorrect identification of patients for carotid endarterectomy, CTA is generally not accepted as an alternative to DSA [6].

CTA in venous sinus occlusive disease

Sinus venous thrombosis often produces unspecific clinical symptoms. Although the combination of seizures, headaches, and focal clinical symptoms are typical in patients with venous sinus occlusive disease (VSOD), there are many patients with other symptoms. In an emergency situation, a quick, available, easy-to-handle method is required to rule out the differential diagnosis of VSOD.

Several studies have shown that CTA has the potential to reliably demonstrate sinus thrombosis. Unlike the CTA technique used in patients with arterial diseases in VSOD, the spiral CT runs from the vertex to the skull and guarantees a high intravenous contrast throughout the whole acquisition. 3-D reconstruction of the dataset is generally not helpful, but evaluation of all axial source images with optimized windowing is necessary (see **Figure 5**).

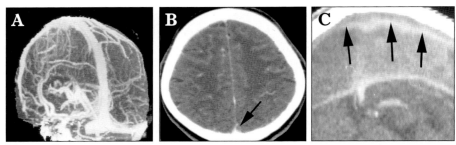

Figure 5. Venous computed tomography-angiography (CTA): normal 3-D angiogram (A). Source image (B) demonstrates empty triangle sign in acute thrombosis of the superior sagittal sinus (black arrow); (C) multiplanar reconstruction in the midline shows the extent of the thrombus (black arrow).

Not all lesions within the enhanced sinus are caused by fresh thrombosis. In addition, intravenous septs and pacchionian granulations can produce sinus opacification. One should be aware of these potential pitfalls. In some cases, it is not possible to differentiate between thrombosis and an abnormality of the sinus by CTA alone; other modalities, such as MRI and MRA, have to be included in the diagnostic work-up. However, in most circumstances, venous CTA has been proven as a quick, easy-to-handle, reliable tool for investigation of the greater venous cerebral system [10].

CTA in acute subarachnoid hemorrhage

CT is the primary imaging tool used in patients with suspected acute subarachnoid hemorrhage (SAH). A 'fresh' SAH is detected by unenhanced CT in >95% of patients. In about 15% of SAH patients, intraparenchymal hemorrhage is also present. Very large hemorrhages or acute hydrocephalus may require an acute surgical intervention to prevent life-threatening herniation. In these cases, CTA can be performed directly after unenhanced CT to demonstrate the location of the aneurysm (see **Figure 6**). In patients with acute SAH, CTA can also enable physicians to plan further patient management. The demonstration of an aneurysm (e.g., basilar-tip aneurysm) that will be treated primarily by an endovascular, as opposed to neurosurgical, approach can result in a one-step angiography under full anesthesia in which the final diagnosis and therapy can be combined (see **Figure 7**). CTA also delivers information about the aneurysm wall: calcifications of the aneurysm or the parent vessel can be demonstrated as well as thrombosis within the aneurysm (see **Figure 8**). This information may have an important influence on any therapeutic discussion [8,11].

However, because of limited spatial resolution, CTA of the circle of Willis only displays aneurysms greater than 2–3 mm. CTA is also limited in its ability to show peripheral aneurysms or aneurysms within or next to the cavernous sinus, and CTA delivers no hemodynamic information, which is essential to plan the therapeutic approach.

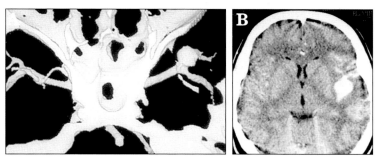

Figure 6. Computed tomography (CT)-angiography in acute rupture of a middle cerebral artery-aneurysm: 3-D angiogram demonstrates the aneurysm (A), while the unenhanced CT-scan shows a space occupying hematoma in the Sylvian fissure (B).

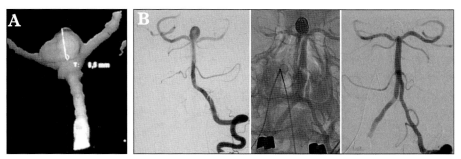

Figure 7. Computed tomography-angiography in basilar-tip-aneurysm: 3-D reconstruction shows aneurysm geometry and allows size measurement of the aneurysm sac (A). This aneurysm was treated with endovascular coiling (B).

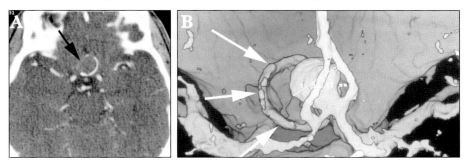

Figure 8. Computed tomography-angiography in a partially thrombosed and calcified aneurysm of the anterior communicating artery. Both thrombus (A – black arrow) and calcification (B – white arrows) are shown in source images and 3-D reconstruction.

MR-angiography

MRA is an MRI study of the vascular structures that produces a 3-D image. It is a noninvasive technique that can be achieved without the need for contrast agents.

Techniques

There are three main MRA techniques available to evaluate vessels: time-of-flight (TOF); phase contrast; and contrast-enhanced.

Time-of-flight MRA

TOF-MRA uses in-flow and flow-through phenomena to increase signals from moving blood while signals from stationary tissue are decreased. Slice thickness can be reduced to 0.7 mm whilst maintaining acceptable acquisition times; however, with the high spatial resolution required, only a small area of interest can be investigated.

TOF-MRA is sensitive to T1-effects; therefore, lesions with short T1 relaxation times are visible on the source images as well as on the 3-D reconstructions. Hence, a hematoma containing methemoglobin will be hyperintense in TOF images and could obscure vascular pathologies (see **Figure 9**). The same is true for thromboses that have been present for some time, they show a very high signal with the TOF technique, and can be misinterpreted as flow. A presaturation band applied above the image volume will suppress venous signal. This is particularly useful when examining areas where arteries and veins are in close proximity (e.g., cavernous sinus).

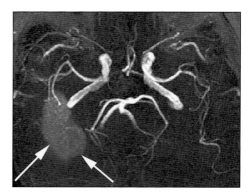

Figure 9. Time-of-flight magnetic resonance angiography in subacute hematoma; methemoglobin within the hematoma (white arrows) overlays middle cerebral artery branches and makes interpretation difficult.

Laminar flow, perpendicular to the imaged volume, is required for ideal images. Artificial signal loss in TOF-MRA is caused by spin saturation in slow flow, or dephasing of spins due to turbulent flow or flow in the plane of volume. These situations occur in hemodynamically relevant stenoses or giant aneurysms, and result in severe overestimation of stenoses or parts of the aneurysm being obscured. However, new interpolation algorithms will allow shorter scan times with increased in-plane and in-slice resolution in the near future [12].

Phase contrast MRA

PC-MRA is essentially a subtraction technique, which relies on phase differences between stationary and moving protons. Background suppression is superior to that of TOF-MRA and problems with hyperintense hemorrhages or fat do not occur in PC-MRA. The major problem with PC-MRA is the long scan time required when high resolution with larger slabs is required. However, this technique is still commonly used to demonstrate flow in the major dural sinuses.

Using a 2-D technique, with velocity encoding ≤15 cm/s, flow within the major cerebral veins can be demonstrated in less than 2 minutes. PC-MRA is also useful in the evaluation of aneurysms after coiling: usually, only small slabs with acceptable scan times are requested, and the significant pitfall of TOF-MRA (thrombosis within the coil package can be misinterpreted as residual flow in the aneurysm) is avoided with PC-MRA [13–15].

Contrast-enhanced MRA

CE-MRA is a new and exciting technique, used increasingly in the evaluation of the greater peripheral vessels. The main advantages of CE-MRA are its short scan time and reduced artifacts due to slow flow and decreased turbulence. However, spatial resolution is still limited with currently available scanners, but this may change in the near future with increased gradient power of the magnetic systems. CE-MRA is already established in the evaluation of cervical vessels, including the origins of the supra-aortic arteries, as an alternative or supplement to ultrasound.

MRA in acute arterial ischemic stroke

With the clinical development of acute stroke MRI protocols, MRA has become a major part of this diagnostic approach. The interpretation of data from diffusion weighted imaging (DWI) and perfusion weighted imaging (PWI) may result in severe pitfalls without adequate information on the status of the circle of Willis. Severe proximal stenoses or occlusion of carotid or vertebral arteries may result in significant changes in brain perfusion due to the recruitment of collaterals. The interpretation of mismatch findings between PWI and DWI must take in to account the findings from MRA to allow a complete vascular and physiologic work-up and early consideration of systemic or local thrombolysis. Usually, a TOF technique with low spatial resolution is used for the stroke MRI protocol to reduce the scan time to less than 3 minutes (see **Figure 10**).

Additional, and often time-consuming, methods to evaluate the cerebral circulation are not necessary to start early treatment. Conventional cerebral angiography must not be performed unless local thrombolysis or another acute endovascular treatment (e.g., emergency stenting) is discussed. In stroke patients

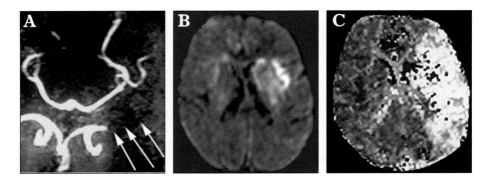

Figure 10. Magnetic resonance imaging in acute left middle cerebral artery-occlusion: time-of-flight magnetic resonance angiography (A) demonstrates vessel occlusion, diffusion-weighted imaging (B) shows areas of abnormal diffusion, and perfusion-weighted imaging (C) shows areas of minor perfusion.

with suspected acute lesions on the extracranial carotids, an additional extracranial MRA can be performed in the same session [16]. This is often possible using the same head coil as for the stroke protocol. In some cases, a head and neck coil is necessary to scan the carotid bifurcation; however, even this procedure with a second positioning of the patient in the scanner can be performed within an acceptable time (<30 minutes). With this technique, acute lesions of the carotid, e.g., carotid dissections, can be diagnosed immediately enabling early commencement of therapy.

MRA in carotid bifurcation stenosis

Doppler sonography is the method of choice to screen for carotid bifurcation stenosis. This technique is popular because it is readily available and inexpensive. However, one of the main criticisms of the technique is operator variability. Another drawback is the inability of this technique to view the distal cervical carotid as well as the aortic arch with the great vessel origins. In patients with a transient ischemic attack (TIA) or stroke, Doppler sonography will exclude those who do not have relevant carotid stenosis. A positive study can then be confirmed with an MRA study. The combination of both studies gives sensitivities and specificities of 95%–100% [17,18].

Selective catheter angiography is performed in <20% of patients during pretreatment evaluation of carotid bifurcation disease. DSA should be performed only in those patients with unclear ultrasound findings or discordance between ultrasound and MRA findings, which occurs in approximately 16% of cases.

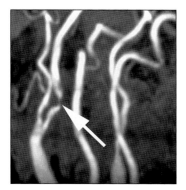

Figure 11. Maximum intensity projection-reconstruction of cervical time-of-flight magnetic resonance angiography demonstrates high-grade internal carotid artery-stenosis on the right (white arrow).

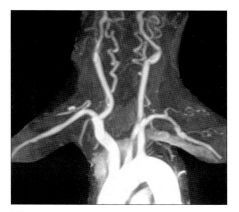

Figure 12. Maximum intensity projection-reconstruction of the aortic arch and the supra-aortic arteries in a contrast-enhanced magnetic resonance angiogram (time of acquisition = 22 seconds). Contrast is injected via the left cubital vein; note the enhancement of the left subclavian vein, the anonymal vein, and pulmonary vessels.

Pretreatment work-up of the craniocervical arteries by MRA should include imaging from the aortic arch to the distal parts of the craniocervical arteries. Additional imaging of the intracranial arteries is recommended to evaluate the whole arterial circulation from the heart to the brain. However, the incidence of relevant proximal or distal tandem stenoses has been quoted as <10% [19].

Until now, 2-D TOF has been the mainstay of MRA to evaluate the carotids (see **Figure 11**). However, with this technique, imaging from the aortic arch to the skull base requires acquisition times of more then 15 minutes, which often results in unacceptable motion artifacts. In addition, TOF-MRA (2-D and 3-D) and PC-MRA often exaggerate the degree of carotid stenoses. More recent studies have shown the value of CE-MRA in the exact evaluation of arterial stenoses.

In contrast to the traditional MRA-techniques, flow turbulence does not play a major role in CE-MRA, because it is not a flow-related but a morphologic imaging technique. Therefore, overestimation of vessel stenoses occurs less often. The acquisition time of the supra-aortic vessels is about 20 seconds in CE-MRA (see **Figure 12**). The timing from start of acquisition to arrival of the contrast bolus is critical to achievement of a high intra-arterial contrast concentration during acquisition in CE-MRA. Appropriate bolus timing can be achieved using a test bolus or an automated bolus detection and scan-triggering scheme. The latter is commercially available on modern scanners.

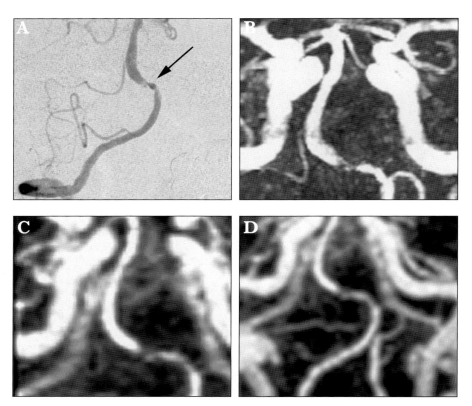

Figure 13. Comparison of different angiographic techniques in symptomatic basilar artery stenosis: intra-arterial digital subtraction angiography (DSA) (A) shows a small ulceration in the stenosis; time-of-flight magnetic resonance angiography (TOF-MRA) (B) overestimates the grade of the stenosis; contrast-enhanced magnetic resonance angiography (CE-MRA) (C) demonstrates the grade of stenosis as compared to that seen with DSA and also shows the ulceration. Image quality increases slightly with a subtracted CE-MRA technique (D).

The use of additional subtraction techniques may increase the signal-to-noise ratio (SNR) but also increase the risk of motion artifacts. The main limitation of CE-MRA of the carotids is the low spatial resolution (see **Figure 13**). The combination of new high-power gradient systems, optimal coil systems and perfect bolus timing increases the spatial resolution of this technique to the sub-millimeter range [20,21]. However, this latest generation of MR scanner will not be widely available for several years.

A combination of TOF-MRA and CE-MRA is the preferred protocol in the pretreatment work-up of patients with suspected carotid stenoses. 2-D TOF-MRA of the carotid bifurcation and the intracranial vessels is used to evaluate those areas with higher spatial resolution and to obtain information about

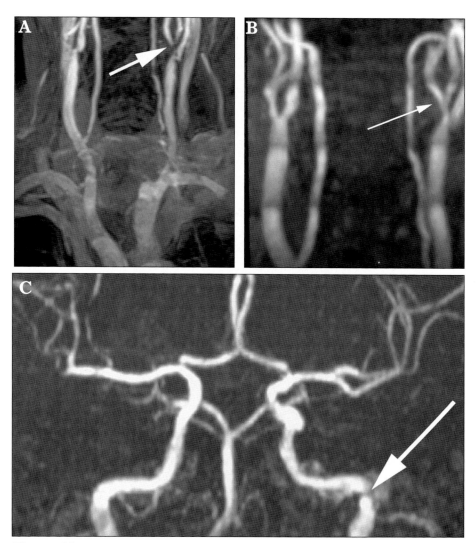

Figure 14. Combined magnetic resonance angiography-protocol in the work-up of symptomatic left internal carotid artery (ICA)-stenosis. Contrast-enhanced MRA (A) demonstrates the aortic arch, supra-aortic situation, and the stenosis of the left carotid bifurcation (white arrow). However, the quality of the supra-aortic area is limited. Time-of-flight (TOF)-MRA (B) of the bifurcation shows left ICA-stenosis more clearly (white arrow). Only intracranial TOF-MRA (C) demonstrates a relevant distal tandem-stenosis of left ICA (white arrow).

the intracranial flow dynamic. CE-MRA is performed to image the aortic arch, the supra-aortic vessels, and the distal extracranial parts. However, even with this protocol, imaging of the origin of the supra-aortic vessels is rarely optimal, and lesions in the carotid siphon are often difficult to evaluate or rule out (see **Figure 14**).

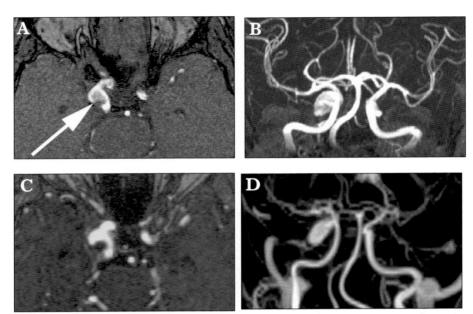

Figure 15. Comparison of time-of-flight magnetic resonance angiography (TOF-MRA) (A, B) and contrast-enhanced magnetic resonance angiography (CE-MRA) (C, D) in a giant intracranial internal carotid artery-aneurysm: in TOF-MRA, flow voids within the aneurysm sac (white arrow) mask the demonstration of the whole aneurysm in source images (A) as well as in maximum intensity projection (MIP) reconstructions (B). The total size of the aneurysm is better demonstrated by CE-MRA (C – source image, D – MIP). However, the spatial resolution is not as good with this technique.

CE-MRA also seems to be an appropriate technique to image giant intra- or extracranial aneurysms because it is less affected by flow-turbulence than other techniques (see **Figure 15**) [22].

MRA in venous sinus occlusive disease
The variety of MRA techniques makes it an ideal tool to evaluate the cerebral venous system. In the emergency situation, thrombosis of the greater sinuses can be ruled out with CTA; however, MRA is the appropriate method to demonstrate the extent of acute thrombosis, to show the extent of venous edema, and to carry out the follow-up in the subacute and chronic stage. Different MR techniques are required to answer different questions in patients with VSOD:

- 2-D PC-MRA is appropriate to demonstrate flow in the superior sagittal sinus (SSS) within a very short scan-time (see **Figure 16**)
- 2-D TOF-MRA is used to demonstrate flow in the transverse sinus and major cortical veins (see **Figure 17**)
- CE 3-D T1-weighted gradient echo sequences or CE-MRA with high spatial resolution are best to show the extent of a thrombus from the SSS into smaller cortical veins (see **Figure 18**)

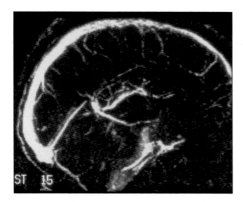

Figure 16. Venous phase contrast magnetic resonance angiography of the superior sagittal sinus and internal veins (time of acquisition = 1.5 minutes).

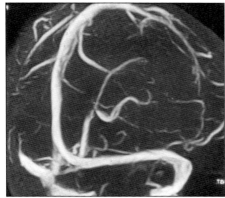

Figure 17. Venous time-of-flight magnetic resonance angiography demonstrates not only the greater cerebral veins, but also the major cortical veins (time of acquisition = 8.5 minutes).

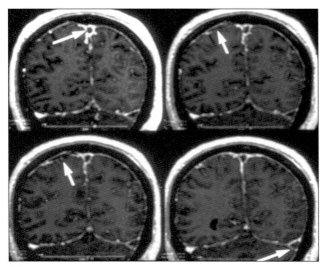

Figure 18. Contrast enhanced high-resolution 3-D T1-weighted gradient-recalled-echo sequence of venous sinus occlusive disease demonstrates thrombus within the superior sagittal sinus, in cortical veins, and in the transversal sinus (white arrows).

In addition to the multiple uses of flow-sensitive MRI, conventional MRI with T1- and T2-weighted sequences is recommended to demonstrate flow voids in the open veins or methemoglobin signaling within the thrombus. A high signal of subacute thrombus, which is older then 3–4 days, may be due to severe pitfalls in flow-sensitive TOF-MRA and may, therefore, be misinterpreted as flow.

MRI is superior to CT in demonstrating the effect of VSOD on the brain parenchyma and should be performed in all patients with proven VSOD. Vasogenic edema is demonstrated with T2-weighted images, DWI can differentiate between vasogenic and cytotoxic edema, and the occurrence of smaller petechial hemorrhages and venous infarcts can be demonstrated by heavily T2*-weighted images [23].

Practical considerations

Intra-arterial DSA is still the gold standard in the imaging of vessels supplying the brain. In comparison to other techniques, DSA shows the greatest spatial resolution and delivers selective hemodynamic information about stenoses and the development of collateral circulation. DSA also provides information on whether or not endovascular treatment of vascular lesions is possible. With the development of 3-D rotational angiography, DSA supplies volume and 3-D information, which benefits the endovascular treatment of intracranial aneurysms and improves the imaging and pretreatment evaluation of extra- and intracranial stenoses.

However, intra-arterial DSA is an invasive method and is associated with morbidity, primarily due to stroke; up to 1% of atherosclerotic patients will develop a stroke, as opposed to ~0.2% of nonatherosclerotic patients [24]. Therefore, intra-arterial DSA should only be performed in those patients in which: other methods are not sufficient (e.g., searching for aneurysms in SAH); non-invasive methods have produced discordant findings; or, the need for endovascular treatment could not be proven.

CTA is widely accepted as an initial vascular screening method in patients with intracranial hemorrhage. In emergency cases, without enough time for performing intra-arterial DSA, CTA can show larger aneurysms or angiomas. CTA is also an ideal instrument to screen acute patients for SSS thrombosis. Modified CTA with an enhanced parenchymal approach is also important in a CT-stroke protocol, when MRI cannot be performed.

MRA, with its variety of techniques, is the second major method of pretreatment work-up in patients with carotid stenoses. The role of MRA in this setting is to confirm the ultrasound-findings. In cases with discordant findings, intra-arterial DSA should be performed. MRA with TOF-technique is a major part of the MRI stroke protocol. The interpretation of DWI and PWI findings should always include the MRA findings to avoid disastrous misinterpretations.

TOF- and PC-MRA are ideal tools to screen patients for aneurysm and to follow-up those who have been treated with an endovascular approach.

Conclusion

Both CTA and MRA will undergo significant developments in the near future and we are likely to see exciting improvements. The recent introduction of multislice CT, and the possible development and clinical use of volume-CT, opens new horizons in the diagnosis of vessel diseases using CT. In addition MRI has also experienced significant changes recently with the introduction of increased gradient powers and the first clinical 3-Tesla scanners. It is impossible to predict which of these noninvasive techniques – CT or MRI – will finally become the gold standard. However, it is certain that one or both will replace conventional DSA as a diagnostic tool.

References

1. Hunter GJ, Hamberg LM, Ponzo JA et al. Assessment of cerebral perfusion and arterial anatomy in hyperacute stroke with three-dimensional functional CT: Early clinical results. *AJNR Am J Neuroradiol* 1998;19:29–37.

2. Wildermuth S, Knauth M, Brandt T et al. Role of CT angiography in patient selection for thrombolytic therapy in acute hemispheric stroke. *Stroke* 1998;29:935–8.

3. Knauth M, Kummer R, Jansen O et al. Potential of CT angiography in acute ischemic stroke. *AJNR Am J Neuroradiol* 1997;18:1001–10.

4. Graf J, Skutta B, Kuhn FP et al. Computed tomographic angiography findings in 103 patients following vascular events in the posterior circulation: Potential and clinical relevance. *J Neurol* 2000;247:760–6.

5. Egelhof T, Jansen O, Winter R et al. CT-angiography in dissection of the internal carotid artery. *Radiologe* 1996;36:850–4.

6. Anderson GB, Ashforth R, Steinke DE et al. CT angiography for the detection and characterization of carotid artery bifurcation disease. *Stroke* 2000;31:2168–74.

7. Sameshima T, Futami S, Morita Y et al. Clinical usefulness of and problems with three-dimensional CT angiography for the evaluation of atherosclerotic stenosis of the carotid artery: Comparison with conventional angiography, MRA, and ultrasound sonography. *Surg Neurol* 1999;51:300–9.

8. Anderson GB, Steinke DE, Petruk KC et al. Computed tomographic angiography versus digital subtraction angiography for the diagnosis and early treatment of ruptured intracranial aneurysms. *Neurosurgery* 1999;45:1315–20; discussion 1320–2.

9. Link J, Brossmann J, Penselin V et al. Common carotid artery bifurcation: Preliminary results of CT angiography and color-coded duplex sonography compared with digital subtraction angiography. *AJR Am J Roentgenol* 1997;168:361–5.

10. Kirchhof K, Jansen O, Sartor K. CT-angiography of cerebral veins. *Fortschr Röntgenstr* 1996;165:232–7. (In German.)

11. Jansen O, Braks E, Hähnel S et al. CT angiography to determine the size of intracranial aneurysms before GDC therapy. *Fortschr Röntgenstr* 1998;169:175–81. (In German.)

12. Chung TS, Joo JY, Lee SK et al. Evaluation of cerebral aneurysms with high-resolution MR angiography using a section-interpolation technique: Correlation with digital subtraction angiography. *AJNR Am J Neuroradiol* 1999;20:229–35.

13. Brunereau L, Cottier JP, Sonier CB et al. Prospective evaluation of time-of-flight MR angiography in the follow-up of intracranial saccular aneurysms treated with Guglielmi detachable coils. *J Comput Assist Tomogr* 1999;23:216–23.

14. Anzalone N, Righi C, Simionato F et al. Three-dimensional time-of-flight MR angiography in the evaluation of intracranial aneurysms treated with Guglielmi detachable coils. *AJNR Am J Neuroradiol* 2000;21:746–52.

15. Derdeyn CP, Graves VB, Turski PA et al. MR angiography of saccular aneurysms after treatment with Guglielmi detachable coils: Preliminary experience. *AJNR Am J Neuroradiol* 1997;18:279–86.

16. Schellinger P, Jansen O, Fiebach J et al. Feasibility and practicality of stroke MRI in hyperacute cerebral ischemia. *AJNR Am J Neuroradiol* 2000;21:1184–9.

17. Sidhu PS, Allan PL. The extended role of carotid artery ultrasound. *Clin Radiol* 1997;52:643–53.

18. De Marco JK, Schonfeld S, Wesbey G. Can noninvasive studies replace conventional angiography in the preoperative evaluation of carotid stenosis? *Neuroimaging Clin N Am* 1996;6:911–29.

19. Brant-Zawadzki M, Heiserman JE. The roles of MR angiography, CT angiography, and sonography in vascular imaging of the head and neck. *AJNR Am J Neuroradiol* 1997;18:1820–5.

20. Remonda L, Heid O, Schroth G. Carotid artery stenosis,occlusion,and pseudo-occlusion: Firstpass,gadolinium-enhanced, three-dimensional MR angiography-preliminary study. *Radiology* 1998;209:95–102.

21. Sardanelli F, Zandrino F, Parodi RC et al. MR angiography of internal carotid arteries: Breath-hold Gd-enhanced 3D fast imaging with steady-state precession versus unenhanced 2D and 3D time-of-flight techniques. *J Comput Assist Tomogr* 1999;23:208–15.

22. Jager HR, Ellamushi H, Moore EA et al. Contrast-enhanced MR angiography of intracranial giant aneurysms. *AJNR Am J Neuroradiol* 2000;21:1900–7.

23. Manzione J, Newman GC, Shapiro A et al. Diffusion- and perfusion-weighted MR imaging of dural sinus thrombosis. *AJNR Am J Neuroradiol* 2000;21:68–73.

24. Grzyska U, Freitag J, Zeumer H. Selective cerebral intraarterial DSA. Complication rate and control of risk factors. *Neuroradiology* 1990;32:296–9.

5

Neurosonology in acute stroke

Stephen Meairs and Fabienne Perren

Introduction

Over three decades ago, continuous-wave (CW) Doppler was introduced as the first neurosonologic method for evaluation of cerebrovascular disease. Since that time, the continuous development of new noninvasive ultrasound techniques has resulted in a variety of clinical applications for assessment of extra- and intracranial arterial diseases. This chapter discusses the clinical merits and limitations of these applications for evaluation of acute stroke. It outlines techniques for identification of stroke etiology and summarizes how neurosonology is used for monitoring of stroke patients. It also addresses the potential utility of new developments in cerebrovascular ultrasound for elucidation of stroke pathophysiology, for improving visualization of arterial disease, and for assessment of cerebral perfusion.

Neurosonologic technology

Doppler sonography

Ultrasound Doppler techniques are commonly used for examining the intra- and extracranial arteries supplying the brain. Interpretation of Doppler signals is based on analysis of the audio signals and of the frequency spectrum. The Doppler effect, named after Christian Doppler who in 1842 described the effect of moving objects on the change in frequency of emitted light, is familiar to anyone who has stood in one place and listened to a source of sound passing by. The pitch of the sound appears to increase as the sound source moves towards the listener, and similarly appears to decrease as the source moves past. Similarly, the Doppler frequency shift, which is the difference between emitted and received ultrasound frequency, is proportional to the velocity of moving blood cells.

CW Doppler systems use two transducers, one of which emits while the other receives ultrasound continuously. While this simple system is easily applicable for the detection of a broad range of flow velocity alterations, including high blood flow velocities associated with severe stenosis, it provides only limited information about the topographic origin of the ultrasound-reflecting source. In contrast, pulse-wave (PW) Doppler systems, in which ultrasound is both emitted and received from a single piezoelectric crystal in the transducer, can provide a depth estimate of the site being insonated. This feature, along with information on the direction of the Doppler frequency shift, is used in transcranial PW-Doppler sonography to locate and differentiate intracranial cerebral arteries.

Doppler ultrasound methods are simple, inexpensive, and noninvasive. In experienced hands, they provide reliable data about hemodynamically significant lumen narrowing. Small lesions, however, cannot be detected by extracranial Doppler sonography alone and information on plaque morphology is not available with this method. CW and PW Doppler are good screening procedures for detection of stenoses and occlusions in the extracranial arteries.

Imaging techniques

Sonographic imaging techniques, such as conventional duplex scanning and color Doppler flow imaging (CDFI), are established routine methods for the evaluation of carotid and vertebral arterial disease. CDFI has also been shown to be of considerable value in transcranial applications. In some neurovascular laboratories, duplex scanning and CDFI are performed in selected patients after CW Doppler sonography, whereas in other centers duplex sonography with Doppler spectrum analysis is directly used for the assessment of extracranial obstructive lesions. Power Doppler imaging (PDI) is another relatively new imaging technique for vascular applications that provides an angiography-like visualization of the arterial lumen.

Several complementary sonographic techniques are available for routine evaluation of the extracranial arteries.

- *B-mode scanning* displays the morphologic features of normal and pathologic vessels [1–4]. Since the extracranial carotid and vertebral arteries lie near the skin, linear array transducers are commonly used at ultrasound frequencies of 7.0–12.0 MHz.

- *Duplex sonography* combines integrated PW Doppler spectrum analysis and B-mode sonography. In addition to providing information about the presence and morphology of arterial lesions, the B-mode image serves as a guide for the placement of the PW Doppler sample volume. Distinct criteria of the Doppler spectrum analysis (see below) are then used to evaluate

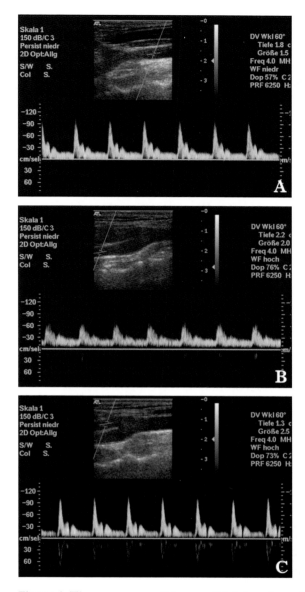

Figure 1. The common carotid artery (A), internal carotid artery (B), and external carotid artery (C) are characterized by distinct Doppler frequency spectrums.

hemodynamics and to categorize carotid artery stenoses. The common, internal, and external carotid arteries (CCA, ICA, and ECA, respectively) are usually characterized by a relatively distinct Doppler frequency spectrum, which allows their identification upon insonation with a PW Doppler system (see **Figure 1**). The emission frequency of the integrated PW Doppler system ranges between 4 and 7 MHz.

- *Color Doppler flow imaging (CDFI)* preserves the advantages of conventional duplex sonography and additionally visualizes color-coded blood flow patterns superimposed on the gray-scale B-mode echotomogram [5–7]. Using a defined color scale, the direction and the average mean velocity of moving blood cells within the sample volume at a given point in time are encoded. Generation of color signals is based on the detection of frequency and phase shifts by means of a multigate transducer. The technique of autocorrelation is used to obtain a *quasi* real-time visualization of color-coded hemodynamics.

- *Power Doppler imaging (PDI)* displays the amplitude of Doppler signals. Color and brightness of the signals are related to the number of blood cells producing the Doppler shift. The greater sensitivity of PDI for detection of blood flow as compared to that of CDFI is due to several factors. Noise can be assigned to a homogenous background, thus allowing the gain to be increased over the level of CDFI. Moreover, in PDI more of the dynamic range of the Doppler signal can be used to increase sensitivity. PDI is also less angle-dependent than CDFI, thus allowing better display of curving or tortuous vessels. Finally, by reliance upon Doppler amplitude, there is no aliasing. This improves display of vessel wall pathology in areas of turbulent flow. First reports on the value of PDI in cerebrovascular ultrasound demonstrated a distinct advantage for assessment of plaque surface structure [8,9]. Since then, this new technique has been further validated as a superior method for characterization of carotid artery plaque surfaces (see **Figure 2**).

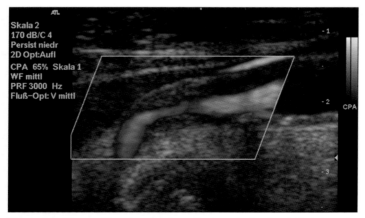

Figure 2. Power Doppler display of stenosis in the left internal carotid artery. Duplex imaging allows simultaneous depiction of homogeneous plaque material.

Identifying extracranial sources of stroke

Carotid artery stenosis

In the initial period of cerebrovascular ultrasound, insonation of the ophthalmic artery was used as an indirect test for detection of significant carotid artery stenosis [10–13]. This periorbital technique still provides useful and rapidly available information regarding the existence of collateral pathways. In the presence of severe stenosis or occlusion of the ICA, retrograde blood supply from the ECA via the ophthalmic anastomosis can be easily detected with CW Doppler. However, with sufficient collateralization from the contralateral carotid or the vertebrobasilar systems, orthograde perfusion of the ophthalmic artery may occur. Accordingly, this indirect test fails to detect hemodynamically significant ipsilateral carotid obstruction in up to 20% of patients. Thus while detection of retrograde perfusion in the ophthalmic artery is a strong indicator of severe pathology within the ipsilateral extracranial carotid system, findings of normal perfusion of the ophthalmic branches cannot exclude severe carotid stenosis or occlusion.

Doppler sonography of the extracranial carotid system is used to detect various degrees of obstruction. According to the distribution of abnormal blood flow patterns within, proximal to, or distal to a narrowed arterial segment, this method provides information on the extent, site, and degree of lesions of more than 40% lumen narrowing. In such lesions the sensitivity (92%–100%) and specificity (93%–100%) of various Doppler techniques have been shown to be similar to those of arteriography [14,15]. Carotid artery plaques producing less than 40% stenosis are usually undetectable by CW and PW Doppler sonography.

Low-frequency PW Doppler devices can be used to assess distal extracranial lesions of the ICA; e.g., carotid dissections, fibromuscular dysplasia, or atypically located atherosclerosis. Adequate positioning of the probe in the submandibular region allows recording of flow velocity in the ICA up to the base of the skull with a recording depth of 50–80 mm.

The degree of carotid obstruction can be defined with Doppler sonography:

1. *Mild stenosis* (40%–60%) is characterized by a local increase in peak and mean flow velocities. Systolic peak velocities range above 120 cm/s (4-MHz probe).

2. *Moderate stenosis* (60%–80%) shows a distortion of normal pulsatile flow in addition to a local increase in peak and mean frequencies. Typically, systolic flow decelerations are found in the poststenotic segment. The systolic peak velocity ranges from 120–240 cm/s.

3. *Severe stenosis* (more than 80%) produces markedly increased peak flow velocities exceeding 240 cm/s and occasionally reaching 500 cm/s. In addition, pre- and poststenotic blood flow velocity is significantly reduced compared with the contralateral unaffected carotid artery. Retrograde flow in the ophthalmic artery may occur.

4. *Subtotal stenosis* (more than 95%) is characterized by variable, usually low peak flow velocities, which decrease once a stenosis becomes pseudo-occlusive. This condition is difficult to separate from complete occlusion and may be misdiagnosed.

5. *ICA Occlusion* is characterized by the absence of any signal along the cervical course of the ICA, while in some cases a low velocity Doppler signal with predominant reversed signal component and absent diastolic flow can be recorded at the presumed origin of the ICA (stump flow). Blood flow velocity in the CCA is reduced, and retrograde perfusion of the ophthalmic artery often occurs.

6. *Severe intracranial obstructions* within the carotid siphon or the middle cerebral artery (MCA) may lead to dampened spectra in the ipsilateral extracranial carotid artery. In addition, alterations of flow direction and signal frequency may occur in the ophthalmic artery depending on the site and degree of the lesion. Intracranial arteriovenous malformations (AVM) and shunts may lead to increased flow velocities in the ipsilateral proximal vessel segments. Therefore, such findings on extracranial Doppler examinations should prompt an appropriate work up for suspected intracranial AVM.

The combination of B-mode imaging and PW Doppler sonography in duplex instruments has considerably improved the accuracy of the noninvasive diagnosis and grading of carotid stenosis. The degree of stenosis can be estimated from distinct parameters of the Doppler frequency spectrum. However, instead of Doppler shift frequencies, equivalent flow velocity values can be obtained after correction of the Doppler insonation angle according to the flow direction in the vessel segment. In CDFI, three sources of information are available for the classification of carotid stenosis: the Doppler frequency spectrum, measurement of the residual vessel lumen, and characteristic color flow patterns.

Doppler frequency spectrum

The time-consuming search for optimal placement of the PW Doppler sample volume is facilitated in CDFI instruments, and reproducibility for the classification of carotid stenosis is significantly improved [16]. Assessment of the

Diameter stenosis (%)	Peak systolic frequency (kHz)	Peak systolic velocity (cm/s)	End diastolic frequency (kHz)	End diastolic velocity (cm/s)
40–60	>4.0	>120	<1.3	<40
61–80	>4.0	>120	>1.3	>40
81–90	>8.0	>240	>3.3	>100

Table 1. Criteria for the classification of internal carotid artery stenosis by pulse-wave Doppler sonography.

Doppler spectrum is particularly important since it can be recorded frequently, even when plaque calcification obscures adequate visualization of color flow patterns and the residual vessel lumen. Using parameters from the Doppler spectrum such as the peak systolic frequency or velocity (see **Table 1**) [16–18], a significantly higher agreement with angiography can be obtained with CDFI than with standard duplex sonography (86.6% vs. 79.6%, respectively, p=0.034). Comparison between color-assisted duplex sonography and planimetry of carotid endarterectomy specimens for the assessment of cross-sectional area reduction revealed a high correlation [19].

Measurement of residual vessel lumen

The methodologic limitations of measurements of residual vessel lumen with B-mode imaging are well documented [20–22]. Using sequential longitudinal and transverse sections, both CDFI and PDI allow more reliable assessment of plaque configuration and relative obstruction by contrasting the intravascular surface [23–27]. Assuming a concentric stenosis, the percentage area reduction in cross-sections is higher than the relative diameter reduction [19]. Early reports on the use of CDFI for evaluation of the degree of stenosis from the relative reduction in the lumen as reflected by the color Doppler flow signal found a relatively poor agreement with angiography on longitudinal (74%) and on transverse (65%) measurements [24]. However, later studies reported a good correlation between transverse lumen reduction on CDFI and diameter reduction on corresponding angiograms of carotid stenosis [27,28]. Measurement of local diameter and area reduction in carotid stenosis can be performed more reliably by PDI than by CDFI due to improved visualization of the residual stenotic lumen [8,9].

Color Doppler flow patterns

Color Doppler flow patterns can provide complementary information for establishing the degree of carotid artery stenosis. Low-grade stenosis (40%–60%) is associated with a relatively long segment of decreased color saturation with absent or minimal post-stenotic turbulence [7]. In moderate obstructions

(61%–80%) the decreased color saturation is more circumscribed, while flow velocity remains high during diastole. Post-stenotic flow is turbulent and flow reversal occurs frequently. High-grade stenosis is characterized by a mosaic pattern (see **Figure 3**) indicating high flow velocity and mixed turbulence [29]. A short segment of maximal color fading or aliasing with severe post-stenotic turbulence and flow reversal provides further evidence for high-grade stenosis [7].

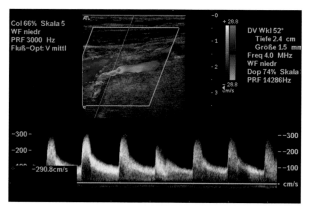

Figure 3. The Doppler spectrum identifies a high-grade stenosis of the carotid artery with maximum peak velocity of 290 cm/s causing left hemispheric stroke. Color Doppler flow imaging demonstrates a mosaic pattern indicating high flow velocity and mixed turbulence.

Although good agreement between angiographic findings and color Doppler flow patterns for low-, middle-, and high-grade stenosis can be obtained [7], several factors can lead to misinterpretation of a semiquantitative analysis of CDFI results. Color-coded hemodynamic patterns are variable due to different plaque configurations and vessel geometries. Interpretation of blue-coded Doppler signals as turbulence, reversed flow, or aliasing phenomena may be difficult in some cases. In addition, peak velocities cannot be directly determined from the color signals since each color pixel on CDFI represents the approximate mean velocity. Other potential color Doppler artifacts include shadowing, reverberation, color bleed, and color noise. In ultrasound systems implementing induced signal amplitude for color suppression, setting the Doppler gain too high or the Doppler reject too low can result in random variations in echo measurements causing hypoechoic regions (e.g., thrombosed vessels) to fill with color. Therefore, it is essential that color Doppler findings be complemented by spectral analysis.

An international consensus meeting has established criteria for the quantification of ICA stenosis [30]. Recommendations were provided for interpretation of maximum Doppler shift velocities, systolic velocity ratios, and residual area.

Plaque morphology

Due to its noninvasive nature, real-time capabilities and general availability, ultrasound has been the most extensively utilized imaging technique for study of carotid artery plaque morphology. High-resolution B-mode imaging alone, and in conjunction with CDFI and PDI techniques, has been used to define parameters for identification of symptomatic or vulnerable plaques. These have included plaque echogenicity, plaque surface structure, and plaque ulcerations.

Carotid artery plaques of homogeneous, moderate intensity echogenicity consist mainly of fibrotic tissue [1,3]. Such plaques rarely show ulceration, perhaps accounting for the lack of a significant correlation between homogeneous echogenicity and the occurrence of focal cerebral ischemia. Heterogeneous plaques represent matrix deposition, cholesterol accumulation, necrosis, calcification, and intraplaque hemorrhage [1,3,4]. Several studies have demonstrated that high-resolution B-mode scanning can characterize echomorphologic features of carotid plaques that correlate with histopathologic criteria [31]. Although echolucent areas within the plaque may represent thrombotic material or hemorrhage, lipid accumulation may produce similar echogenicity [32].

Plaque calcification produces acoustic shadowing. Depending on the location of the plaque and on the extent of calcification, acoustic shadowing can be a major obstacle for adequate ultrasonographic visualization. Initial studies of plaque echogenicity with B-mode ultrasound reported an association between heterogeneous plaques and the occurrence of cerebrovascular events [33–37]. Support for this association was provided by several investigations of endarterectomy specimens which suggested a correlation between intraplaque hemorrhage and transient ischemic attacks and stroke [38–41]. Later studies, however, were unable to confirm these observations [42–44].

Whether or not differences in plaque echogenicity can distinguish between symptomatic and asymptomatic plaques continues to be a debatable subject. More recent ultrasonographic studies have renewed the notion that heterogeneous carotid plaques are more often associated with intraplaque hemorrhage and neurologic events, and conclude that evaluation of plaque morphology may be helpful in selecting patients for carotid endarterectomy [45–47]. Others argue that lipid-rich plaques are more prone to rupture and suggest that an association between intraplaque hemorrhage and a high lipid content, as revealed in B-mode ultrasound, may support this theory [48]. These newer findings have been negated by other research groups finding little correlation between plaque morphology and histological specimens [49]. A definitive study on the significance of heterogeneous plaque structure found no differences in volume of intraplaque hemorrhage, lipid core, necrotic core, or plaque calcification in patients with highly stenotic carotid lesions undergoing endarterectomy, regardless of preoperative symptom status [50].

Attempts to characterize plaque surface structure with B-mode ultrasound have been disappointing. Although a relatively good differentiation between smooth, irregular, and ulcerative plaque surfaces has been obtained for postmortem carotid artery specimens [3], the *in vivo* accuracy as compared to findings at carotid endarterectomy has been considerably poorer [16,31,49,51]. Commonly used parameters for identification of plaque ulceration have been surface defects showing a depth and length of ≥2 mm with a well-defined base in the recess [15]. Using these criteria, B-mode imaging has failed to provide a satisfactory diagnostic yield for ulcerative plaques, with a sensitivity of only 47% [31]. Other groups have been unable to distinguish between the presence or absence of intimal ulcerations with B-mode scans [52]. Diagnostic sensitivity for detection of plaque ulceration with ultrasound is affected by the degree of carotid stenosis and increases to 77% in plaques associated with 50% or less stenosis [31].

Whether plaque surface irregularities or ulcerations are useful parameters for defining patients at risk for carotid embolism remains unclear. Advocates of a pathophysiologic relationship maintain that ulcerations represent fertile ground for potential thrombosis and consequent embolic events. This contention is supported by studies demonstrating an association between angiographically defined ulcerations and an increased risk of stroke in medically treated symptomatic patients [53]. In spite of the poor sensitivity and specificity of arteriography for detection of plaque ulceration [31], it should be remembered that many ulcers are smooth and thick, containing no thrombus at all for putative plaque embolism [54]. Moreover, pathologic studies have shown that in asymptomatic carotid plaques with stenosis exceeding 60%, there is an increased frequency of plaque hemorrhages, ulcerations, and mural thrombi, as well as numerous healed ulcerations and organized thrombi [55]. Likewise, comparisons of symptomatic and asymptomatic large, stenotic carotid endarterectomy plaques have revealed a high incidence of complex plaque structure and complications in each [42,56]. There appears, therefore, to be little difference in plaque constituents or plaque surface structure between specimens from symptomatic and asymptomatic patients. These findings suggest that a simple description of plaque structure or an identification of plaque ulceration as depicted in current clinical imaging techniques, i.e., ultrasound, MRI and angiography, may be of doubtful significance for predicting the vulnerability of carotid plaques.

Occlusion and pseudo-occlusion of the carotid artery

The diagnosis of carotid occlusion by B-mode echotomography alone without Doppler sonography is not reliable since the residual vascular lumen frequently cannot be visualized adequately in complicated heterogeneous, partially calcified, high-grade obstructions. In acute thrombotic occlusion, echolucent material fills the vascular lumen, which can hardly be differentiated on the gray-scale from blood flow in a patent ICA. CW Doppler and duplex sonography have a significantly higher accuracy for the diagnosis of ICA occlusion; however, the differentiation from a subtotal stenosis remains difficult. The PW Doppler spectrum and color signals in ICA occlusion typically demonstrate a marked reduction of the systolic and diastolic blood flow velocity in the CCA and an internalized ECA with high diastolic flow velocity indicating collateral supply via the ophthalmic artery. Color-coded intravascular Doppler signals are absent in the occluded ICA; however, blue-coded flow reversal in the residual stump at the bifurcation (stump flow) may occur. The capacity of modern CDFI and PDI instruments to detect very slow blood flow velocities has markedly improved the sensitivity for the diagnosis of a subtotal ICA stenosis and pseudo-occlusion, which may represent candidates for vascular surgery.

CCA occlusion is a relatively rare condition that can be reliably diagnosed by conventional duplex sonography and CDFI [57,58]. It is important to assess whether the ICA distal to the CCA occlusion is patent, since this is a prerequisite for surgical intervention [59–62]. CDFI typically displays blue-coded signals in the ECA due to reversed flow direction and orthograde filling of the ICA in the absence of Doppler signals in the CCA.

Carotid artery dissection

Ultrasound is useful for diagnosis of carotid artery dissection, a cause of transient or permanent neurologic deficits, particularly in young patients. ICA dissection usually occurs spontaneously and results in a typical syndrome of focal cerebral deficits, headache, neck pain, and ipsilateral Horner's syndrome.

Various patterns can be observed in carotid dissection. CDFI can show marked flow reversal at the origin of the ICA in systole and absent or minimal blood flow in diastole corresponding to a high-resistance bidirectional Doppler signal [63]. B-mode scans can demonstrate a tapered lumen and occasionally a floating intimal flap [64]. Narrowing of the true lumen by the false lumen thrombus can be associated with a low velocity Doppler waveform. The direction of flow in a patent false lumen can vary from being forward, reversed or bidirectional. The flow dynamics in carotid dissections are complex and are primarily dependent upon the presence of thrombus within the false lumen, the entry and exit flaps if the false lumen is patent, the motion of the flap wall, and the extent of the dissection [65]. In some patients the only finding may be a retromandibular high-velocity signal associated with a distal stenosis of the cervical carotid artery [66].

Follow-up examinations of carotid dissections demonstrate gradual normalization of the Doppler spectrum, indicating recanalization of the ICA within a few weeks to months in more than two-thirds of patients [67]. Carotid aneurysms can occur as complications of ICA dissections. Their follow-up with angiography and magnetic resonance angiography/imaging (MRA/MRI) can be complemented with ultrasonography due to development of broadband transducers with improved axial resolution and depth penetration [68].

Vertebral artery stenosis and occlusion

Examination of the vertebral artery with ultrasound is limited to its origin from the subclavian artery, the proximal pretransverse segment, short intertransverse segments between the third and sixth cervical vertebrae, and to the atlas loop. Although PW Doppler criteria for vertebral artery stenosis are similar to those used for diagnosis of carotid artery stenosis and have been defined by several duplex studies, classification and detection of vertebral artery stenosis or occlusion is more difficult than in the carotid arteries [69–71]. One reason for this difficulty is that variations in arterial caliber are frequent in vertebral arteries. Numerous collateral pathways of the vertebral system can permit orthograde flow to the basilar artery even in the face of vertebral occlusion. These features make examination of the vertebral artery at several locations mandatory. CDFI allows noninvasive quantification of flow in the vertebral artery system in more than 95% of all patients [72] and facilitates identification of the proximal segment and ostium, the predominant location of extracranial vertebral stenosis, and the atlas loop [73,74]. Using this technique, normal flow velocities of the vertebral artery origin (V_0 segment), the pre- (V_1 segment), and the intertransverse (V_2 segment) have been recently documented [75].

Correct interpretation of Doppler results from the vertebral artery requires knowledge of Doppler parameters from both the contralateral vertebral artery and from the carotid system. For example, an increase in the systolic or diastolic velocity profile of the proximal vertebral artery, although suggestive of stenosis, can also occur as a compensatory response to a variety of conditions of the contralateral vertebral artery such as hypoplasia, aplasia, stenosis, or occlusion, and to severe obstruction of the carotid system.

The predominant site of extracranial vertebral artery stenosis is the ostium of the subclavian artery. The atlas loop (V_3) and intracranial (V_4) segment are involved less frequently, and stenoses in the intertransverse segments are rare. A peak systolic frequency exceeding 4 kHz assessed by means of the integrated PW Doppler system indicates a relevant vertebral stenosis. Features of color-coded Doppler signals correspond to those of carotid stenosis. With an increasing degree of luminal narrowing, decreased color saturation becomes more circumscribed and turbulence and post-stenotic flow reversal are more severe. Hemodynamically significant obstruction of the intracranial vertebral artery produces a high-resistance Doppler waveform with a resistivity index exceeding 0.80 [74]. However, the Doppler spectrum may be normal if flow to the ipsilateral posterior inferior cerebellar artery is preserved. In acute proximal vertebral artery occlusion PW Doppler spectra cannot be recorded and color Doppler signals are absent in the pre- and intertransverse segments. However, demonstration of the vascular lumen differentiates this condition from vertebral hypoplasia, defined in pathoanatomical studies as a decrease in vascular lumen diameter below 2 mm [76].

Vertebral artery dissection

Vertebral artery dissection is one of the most common causes of brainstem strokes in young patients [77,78]. It presents with neck pain, occipital headache, and signs and symptoms of brainstem or cerebellar ischemia in about 90% of patients, and commonly leaves a permanent deficit [79–81]. The role of ultrasound in diagnosis of vertebral artery dissection remains uncertain. In contradistinction to carotid artery dissection there is no pathognomonic ultrasound finding for vertebral artery dissection if the lesion affects the V_2–V_4 segments. Examination of the atlas loop can show absent, low bidirectional, or low post-stenotic flow signals [82]. In dissections of the V_1 segment, the stenotic segment can be identified directly, while absent flow in the intertransverse segments should similarly raise the question of vertebral dissection. Further findings can include a localized increase in the diameter of the artery with hemodynamic signs of stenosis or occlusion at the same level, decreased pulsatility, and the presence of intravascular echoes in the enlarged segment [83,84]. Occasionally an intramural hematoma is found [85].

Transcranial Doppler (TCD) can be helpful in determining the length of dissection [86]. The combined use of extracranial Doppler, TCD, and duplex sonography increases the diagnostic yield to detect vertebral artery dissection. Consideration of any abnormal sonographic finding resulted in a yield of 86%, whereas reliance upon definite abnormal findings (absent flow signal, severely reduced flow velocities, absent diastolic flow, bidirectional flow, or stenosis signal) reduced the diagnostic yield to only 64% [82]. Similar results were obtained in another study in which ultrasound abnormalities (high-resistance signal, occlusion, and bilateral retrograde flow) were found in eight of ten vertebral artery dissections [87]. Detection of abnormal flow patterns in the vertebral artery in cases of suspected dissection may guide further diagnostic imaging procedures and therapeutic measures. However, since unremarkable ultrasound findings do not exclude the diagnosis of vertebral dissection, further work-up in these cases is mandatory.

The role of transcranial Doppler in evaluation of stroke

TCD uses high-energy bidirectional pulsed Doppler, typically at a low frequency of 2 MHz, for intracranial vascular examination via transtemporal, transorbital, and transnuchal bone windows. Applications for TCD in stroke imaging include detection of intracranial stenosis and occlusion, evaluation of intracranial collateral circulations, detection of vasospasm in subarachnoid hemorrhage (SAH), and assessment of cerebral autoregulation. TCD monitoring techniques are available for detection of high intensity transient signals suggestive of microembolism and for surveillance of intracranial hemodynamics during stroke therapy. The introduction of transcranial CDFI (TCDFI) has led to greater accuracy in vessel identification, and reports on the merits of CDFI for detection of cerebral aneurysms, evaluation of AVM, and characterization of vessel morphology are now available. More recent technologic advances have enhanced the capabilities of TCD ultrasonography. These include transcranial power Doppler, contrast-enhanced CDFI, 3-D transcranial power Doppler angiography, and contrast harmonic perfusion imaging.

With conventional TCD, intracranial basal arteries are identified by flow direction, depth of the Doppler sample volume, and probe position. Since flow velocities of intracranial vessels are known to vary with age and sex [88], hematocrit [89], and end-tidal CO_2 partial pressure, a standardized TCD examination procedure is mandatory [90]. Normal values of flow velocities of the basal cerebral arteries have been determined in several studies [14,91–96]. Optimal performance and correct interpretation of TCD studies require knowledge of the clinical setting and of results from extracranial ultrasound examinations.

TCDFI facilitates identification of basal cerebral arteries [97]. While conventional TCD sonography assumes a 0-degree Doppler angle for the calculation of flow velocities, TCDFI allows correction for the Doppler insonation angle. The magnitude of the angle of insonation and the effect on flow velocity estimates in intracranial vessels have been determined through visually controlled measurements of the Doppler angle of insonation made by color flow imaging: angle-corrected peak systolic flow velocities were 3%–30% higher as compared to uncorrected velocity readings by conventional Doppler sonography [98]. Similar findings were reported in another study: in 14.5% the angle-corrected velocity was

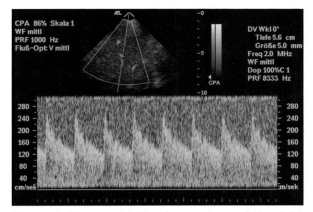

Figure 4. Transcranial Doppler spectrum of the right middle cerebral artery from a patient suffering from right hemispheric transient ischemic attacks. Maximum peak velocity of 260 cm/s is consistent with a moderate to high-grade stenosis.

25%–50% higher and in 10.8% it was more than 50% higher as compared to the uncorrected velocity [99]. Although TCDFI is considered by many to be the ultrasonic method of choice in evaluation of the intracranial circulation, there are no data on the failure rate of TCDFI in a large group of patients.

Intracranial stenosis and occlusion

Significant narrowing of intracranial arteries results in localized increases in mean and peak flow velocities, turbulence and reversed flow phenomena, and reduction of pre- or post-stenotic flow velocities [100–102]. Stenosis of greater than 50% lumen narrowing (see **Figure 4**) can be reliably detected in arterial segments with anatomically favorable insonation angles such as the M_1 segment of the MCA and the P_1 segment of the posterior cerebral artery (PCA).

A reliable diagnosis of occlusion in the M_1 segment can only be made when unequivocal evidence of blood flow in the ipsilateral anterior cerebral artery (ACA) or PCA can be obtained, thus differentiating this condition from high ultrasound attenuation and poor echo window insonation. Further findings supporting MCA occlusion are dampened spectra in segments proximal to the occlusion, reversed flow direction in distal MCA branches, and abnormally elevated ipsilateral ACA flow velocities [103]. In a series of 467 patients, the sensitivity for the detection of MCA occlusion by TCD was 79% with a specificity of 100% [104]. Contrast-enhanced TCDFI (CE-TCDFI) may be more accurate than TCD in demonstrating occlusions of the MCA [105] and is particularly useful in cases of inadequate bone windows [106]. A recent multicenter clinical trial demonstrated that TCDFI is a feasible, fast, and valid noninvasive bedside method for evaluating the MCA in an acute stroke setting, particularly when contrast enhancement is applied [107].

TCD examinations of the vertebrobasilar arteries are less reliable than those of the anterior circulation. The junction of the basilar artery is difficult to define by TCD criteria alone, and investigation of the entire course of the basilar artery, usually limited by excessive insonation depth with poor signal to noise ratio [108], can be achieved in only 30% of patients. As in the anterior circulation, partial obstructions are easier to detect than total occlusion. Using intra-arterial digital subtraction angiography as a standard reference, TCD has demonstrated sensitivities of 74%–87% and specificities of 80%–86% for detection of large vessel occlusive disease of the intracranial vertebrobasilar system [109,110]. Best results, however, are obtained when TCD is used in combination with cerebral angiography [108] or MRA [111]. Unfortunately, detection of basilar artery occlusion is poor with a sensitivity of only 36% [112]. This is of major clinical importance in evaluation of patients suspected of suffering from acute basilar artery thrombosis.

Assessment of intracranial collateralization

The presence of intracranial collateralization in patients with stenosis or occlusion of the extracranial carotid arteries can be investigated with conventional TCD. Findings compatible with collateral flow over the anterior communicating artery include retrograde flow in the ipsilateral ACA, increased peak and mean velocities in both ACAs, increased velocities and low frequency signals in the midline indicating functional stenosis of the anterior communicating artery, and decreased MCA velocity during contralateral CCA compression. Collateralization from the posterior circulation is suggested by increased velocities in the ipsilateral P_1 segment of the PCA or in the basilar artery as well as by low frequency signals in the posterior communicating artery. Leptomeningeal anastomosis, although more difficult to assess, may be associated with increased velocities in proximal and distal segments of the PCA and with retrograde flow signals in distal MCA branches. TCD can also detect retrograde flow in the ophthalmic artery, another avenue for collateralization.

Flow velocities in the MCA distal to significant stenosis and occlusion vary with regard to the efficacy of intracranial collateralization. Whereas reduced MCA velocities and pulsatility indexes have been found ipsilateral to symptomatic carotid occlusion [113,114], normal peak and mean velocities indicating adequate collateralization have been reported for asymptomatic patients [115].

Microembolic signal detection

Stemming from his early work in 1969 on transcutaneous ultrasonographic detection of air bubbles evoked by decompression [116], Spencer described a novel application of TCD for detection of MCA emboli during carotid

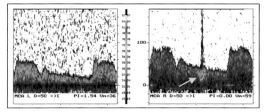

Figure 5. Simultaneous transcranial Doppler monitoring of high intensity transient signals in the left (left image) and right (right image) middle cerebral artery (MCA). Note the high intensity signal (arrow) occurring in the right MCA, presumably of microembolic origin.

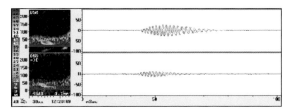

Figure 6. Multigate Doppler technique for improved identification of microemboli. Here the middle cerebral artery is insonated simultaneously at two locations. The delay in time between the appearance of high intensity signals at the two gates is strong evidence for a microembolic particle (an artifact would appear simultaneously at both gates).

endarterectomy [117]. Subsequent studies confirmed the ability of TCD to detect high intensity transient signals (HITS) corresponding to both gaseous and solid microembolic materials during procedures such as angiography [118,119], carotid angioplasty [120], open heart surgery [121,122], and carotid endarterectomy [123,124], as well as in patients with transient ischemic attacks or stroke [125-128], asymptomatic carotid stenosis [129], heart valve prosthesis [130,131], and intracranial arterial disease [132].

Definition of HITS
HITS are usually visualized in the fast Fourier transform (FFT). Using this signal analysis approach, three criteria for defining a HITS were proposed by a consensus committee [133] in 1995: 1) duration is less than 300 ms, 2) exceeds the background by at least 3 dB, and 3) is unidirectional within the Doppler velocity spectrum. HITS detection can be performed by insonating any of the three major vessels of the circle of Willis, although monitoring of the carotid arteries [134] and the jugular veins has also been reported [135]. In most cases, the main stem of the MCA is insonated with a 2-MHz probe using the temporal bone window (see **Figure 5**). Sophisticated multigate techniques have been developed that interrogate two sample volumes along a vessel to enable better differentiation between artifacts and moving particles (see **Figure 6**).

The interobserver agreement for the detection of HITS is high [136–138], with kappa values of ~0.95. Unfortunately, this technique is very time consuming. Although HITS monitoring of several hours' duration could potentially increase the yield of HITS in situations where they occur with relatively low frequency or high variability, this is not practical in routine applications. A number of research groups have addressed this problem by developing automated systems for HITS detection. However, none of these has the required sensitivity and specificity for clinical use [139]. Whether new signal analysis techniques such as simultaneous insonation with two frequencies, e.g., 1 and 2 MHz [140], nonlinear forecasting [141], the recognition of specific postembolic spectral patterns [142], or the application of the narrow band hypothesis [143] can illuminate specific properties of HITS will be a matter of further research.

Localizing the source of embolism in stroke patients
Results on the frequency of HITS suggestive of microemboli from the heart or from the proximal arteries of the intracranial circulation have been variable [144,145]. In patients with heart valve prosthesis, thousands of clinically silent events can be recorded whereas in patients with symptomatic carotid stenoses, HITS are relatively rare events. It appears that emboli of cardiac and carotid origin may have different ultrasonic characteristics, which are likely related to composition and size [146]. The clinical relevance of these features, however, is unclear.

Following the report of HITS during carotid endarterectomy [117], similar signals occurring spontaneously were recognized in patients with symptomatic carotid artery disease [125,127,129]. Since the microembolic signals (MES) disappeared after carotid endarterectomy [126,147,148], it was assumed that the atherosclerotic carotid plaque had been the source of the MES. In an unselected group of stroke patients examined within 1 month after cerebral infarction, the prevalence of ipsilateral MES in the largest series published was approximately 10% [149]. If the interval following the acute event is shorter, the prevalence of MES may increase. TCD monitoring within 2 days after admission showed that approximately 25% of an unselected patient group were positive [150]. Patients with a carotid stenosis of at least 40% have been reported to have significantly more MES (39%) than those without a carotid stenosis (18%). Similarly, the prevalence of MES in a comparable group of patients was reported to approach 50% when monitoring was performed immediately after admission, and 1 and 2 days thereafter [151]. Of the studied group, 44% had a carotid stenosis or occlusion and 62% of these were MES-positive.

Apart from the role of examination timing in determining the likelihood of detecting MES in symptomatic carotid artery disease [147,152,153], the degree of carotid stenosis may correlate with the number of measured MES, i.e., the more severe the narrowing, the more MES are detected [151,154,155]. Interestingly, complete carotid occlusion has been found to be associated with a high MES count [155]. Contrary to the preceding discussion on the doubtful relevance of plaque ulcerations in pathoanatomical studies, other studies maintain a relationship between preoperative MES count and carotid plaque ulceration [156]. Similarly, HITS monitored in the middle cerebral arteries of patients with carotid stenosis have been reported to correlate with the appearance of ipsilateral plaque ulceration [157].

There is some evidence that HITS detected during the dissection phase of carotid endarterectomy may correlate with clinically silent infarctions demonstrated with MRI [123]. Moreover, in a few cases, a relationship between persistent particulate embolization in the immediate postoperative period and both incipient carotid artery thrombosis and the development of major neurologic deficits [124] has been observed. In carotid angioplasty, embolization at the time of intervention is very common but usually asymptomatic. Late embolization, occurring in a minority of patients, may account for the small but significant risk of delayed stroke [120].

Carotid dissections can cause neurologic deficits either by hemodynamic or embolic mechanisms. As anticoagulants are often used in this setting to prevent neurologic deterioration and stroke recurrence, it would be valuable to differentiate between the two mechanisms. HITS detection would seem an ideal technique for this purpose. Reports on the relationship between MES and the clinical or imaging features of carotid dissection, however, have been conflicting. While one study of patients with carotid dissections [158] reported that the detection of HITS had no clinical significance, another investigation found that MES occurrence on serial TCD monitoring was associated with an increased risk of early ischemic recurrence [159]. Further studies will be necessary to settle this issue.

Microembolism can also occur in giant cell arteritis [160]. Similarly, MES may be related to disease activity in systemic lupus erythematosus with antiphospholipid syndrome [161].

HITS occur predominantly in patients with large vessel territory stroke patterns and persisting deficits, most likely due to artery-to-artery or cardiogenic embolism [149]. In contrast, patients with small vessel disease only occasionally present with HITS. Thus, the detection of HITS may support the classification of the individual pathogenesis of cerebral ischemia, in particular when multiple risk constellations for stroke coexist. Moreover, detection of recurrent microembolic events by TCD monitoring can provide useful guidance for pathophysiologically oriented treatment of stroke patients [162].

Predicting early recurrence of ischemia

TCD-detected microemboli in stroke patients may be associated with an increased prevalence of prior cerebrovascular ischemia [152,155], thus suggesting a role of MES as a risk factor for cerebral ischemia. Asymptomatic carotid stenoses are associated with MES, but to a much lesser extent than symptomatic stenoses [148,154,163,164]. Studies addressing early recurrent ischemic events after stroke or TIA in patients with a carotid stenosis [165,166] have found the presence of MES to be a predictor for early ischemic recurrence.

Relationship between MES and brain damage

In the majority of cases where HITS are detected, it remains unclear whether these phenomena are associated with an increased risk of functional or morphologic brain damage [167]. This problem has been compounded by the wide variety of parameters used by different investigators for MES detection. A Consensus Group on Microembolus Detection has reported guidelines for the proper use of TCD microembolism detection in clinical practice and scientific investigations [168]. They suggested that technical instruments (ultrasound device, transducer size and type, FFT size, FFT length, FFT overlap, high-pass filter settings), methodology (identification of arteries insonated, insonation depth, detection threshold, scale settings, axial extension of sample volume, recording time) and methods for analysis and interpretation (algorithms for signal intensity measurement, standardization of inter- and intra-observer variability, comparison of semi-automatic embolus detection algorithms) be reported and validated in each individual laboratory to establish the required sensitivity and specificity for clinical use and scientific application.

Venous thrombosis

TCD methods can also be used to evaluate the basal cerebral veins, which can be identified based on their anatomic relation to specific arteries [169]. As in other applications, power- and frequency-based color-coded duplex sonography aids in the assessment of cerebral veins and sinuses [170]. Recently, standardized protocols for intracranial venous examinations and reference data for clinical applications have been described [171].

There is evidence suggesting that TCD can detect and monitor intracranial venous hemodynamics and collateral pathways in patients with confirmed cerebral venous thrombosis [172,173]. TCDFI appears to allow a more reliable evaluation of the major deep cerebral veins and posterior fossa sinuses in cases of sinus thrombosis. The anterior and mid portions of the superior sagittal sinus and cortical veins, however, cannot be assessed [174]. Here, increased venous blood flow velocity can be used as an indirect criterion for indicating a cerebral venous thrombosis. Superior evaluation of transverse sinus thrombosis can be obtained by using echo contrast agents (see below) [175]. Further prospective studies are necessary to establish the sensitivity and specificity of neurosonologic techniques for diagnosis and monitoring of intracranial venous thrombosis.

Dolichoectatic arteries and intracranial vasculopathies

Noninvasive diagnosis of intracranial dolichoectatic arteries [176], a cause of transient ischemic attacks or stroke [177], can be achieved with TCD in combination with computed tomography (CT) or MRI. The dramatic reductions in peak and mean flow velocities that are often observed in these patients suggest a thromboembolic mechanism of ischemia in slow flow territories. TCD is also sensitive and specific for the detection of arterial vasculopathy in sickle cell disease [178,179] and has been used for assessment of reversible multisegmental narrowing of cerebral arteries in postpartum cerebral angiopathy [180].

Detection of right-to-left cardiac shunts

Paradoxical embolism through a patent foramen ovale (PFO) is a known cause of embolic stroke and transient ischemic attack in patients with stroke of uncertain etiology. TCD monitoring of the basal intracranial vessels during intravenous injection of contrast media can be used for the detection of right-to-left shunts, e.g., PFO, by documentation of microbubbles reaching the brain [181–183]. TCD results correlate well with those of transesophageal echocardiography (TEE) when a standardized procedure including the Valsalva maneuver is used [184].

Of considerable interest are reports on the variability of the detection of PFO when using different examination techniques. For example, the sensitivity of diagnosing PFO with both TCD and TEE is considerably higher when contrast media is injected into the femoral vein rather than into the antecubital vein, the current route for contrast media application [185]. This may be related to different inflow patterns to the right atrium because inferior vena caval flow is directed to the right atrial septum and superior vena caval flow to the tricuspid valve. The timing of the Valsalva maneuver, the dose of the contrast medium, and the patient's posture during the examination are further factors influencing detection of PFO [186].

Echocontrast studies in stroke diagnosis

The ability of intravenous contrast media to increase the echogenicity of flowing blood has been known for some time [187]. Only recently, however, has there been an increasing demand for use of echo-enhancing agents in assessment of cerebrovascular disease (e.g., transcranial ultrasound studies in patients with severe hyperostosis of the skull, quantification of internal carotid stenosis in the presence of calcification, differentiation between internal carotid occlusion and pseudo-occlusion, assessment of intracranial aneurysms and AVM, and investigation of the basilar and intracranial vertebral arteries).

Commercially available contrast agents consist of microbubbles with average diameters from 3 µm to 6 µm in concentrations typically in the order of 10^8 microbubbles/mL. The microbubbles are normally stabilized against dissolution by surfactants, phospholipids, or a surface layer of partially denatured albumin. They offer an opportunity to obtain anatomical and physiologic information beyond that provided by current ultrasound imaging and Doppler systems. Among other applications, today's agents can enhance the ultrasound signal by 10 dB to 30 dB [188], enabling the detection of flow in deeper and smaller vessels.

The first generation of ultrasound contrast agents consisted of air-filled microbubbles. Examples of such agents are Albunex® (Molecular Biosystems Inc., San Diego, CA), which is produced by controlled sonication of a 5% human serum albumin solution, and Levovist® (Schering AG, Berlin, Germany), which is a galactose-based agent stabilized by 0.01% palmitic acid. Albunex is approved by the Food and Drug Administration (FDA) for use in the United States, and Levovist is approved for use in Europe. However, because of the low concentration of air gases in the systemic circulation, the air contained inside these agents quickly diffused out of the microbubbles after injection into the body [189]. The type of gas inside the bubble determines the dwell time in the circulation [190], and can also affect the backscattered signal in both linear and nonlinear regimes [191]. Thus, a second generation of ultrasonic agents was formed consisting of microbubbles containing less soluble gases, such as perfluorocarbons or sulfur hexafluoride.

Carotid stenosis

Clinical studies with Levovist have shown it to be safe and effective in improving diagnostic confidence for patients with carotid artery stenosis. Contrast enhancement helps to reduce operator variability, improves ultrasound images, and can aid in distinguishing between pseudo and true occlusions, thus helping to identify patients who will benefit most from surgery [192]. First reports on the use of ultrasonic contrast media to investigate carotid arteries demonstrated a significant improvement in characterization and quantification of severe internal carotid stenosis [193]. In further studies, Levovist considerably improved image quality in patients with high-grade carotid stenosis and allowed better visualization of the entire length of the intrastenotic residual flow lumen, suggesting echo contrast media might play an important role in the diagnosis of

ICA occlusion [194]. Recent data suggest that PDI without contrast agents may approach the diagnostic yield achieved with the combined approach for assessment of carotid artery pseudo-occlusion [195]. Although contrast agents will continue to play an important role in ultrasonographic evaluation of high-grade carotid stenosis, further studies will be necessary to define the clinical setting in which their use is mandatory.

Insufficient transcranial bone windows

In TCD sonography, insonation through the transtemporal bone window is often impaired by an insufficient signal-to-noise ratio, especially in elderly patients. Echo contrast agents have been shown to provide conclusive transcranial examinations in most patients with insufficient ultrasound penetration. Most studies have been performed with the galactose-based microbubble agent Levovist. Depending on the concentration of Levovist, the average maximal transcranial signal enhancement is approximately 12.0 ± 5.4 dB for 300 mg/mL [196]. Similarly, Albunex has been shown to improve the quality of TCD examinations through better visualization of the ICA, the MCA, and the circle of Willis [197], although the relatively short duration of the contrast enhancement is a limiting factor.

Contrast agents have also been shown to enhance diagnoses when using TCDFI in patients with poor tissue penetration where imaging of vessels would otherwise be inadequate [198]. Other studies have confirmed these initial findings in patients whose basal arteries could not be assessed adequately with transcranial CDFI. After administration of Levovist, over 85% of examinations of the MCA, the ACA, the P_1 and P_2 segments of the PCA, and the supraclinoid portion of the ICA siphon were satisfactory [199]. Moreover, use of intravenous contrast material often enables the entire circle of Willis to be evaluated from a single temporal-bone acoustic window when using both PDI and CDFI [200]. Recently, contrast agents have been used to enable intracranial insonation through lateral and paramedian frontal bone windows, thus offering a new approach to study the circle of Willis, the venous midline vasculature, and the frontal parenchyma [201]. The technical success rate of 3-D transcranial PDI investigations has also been improved with contrast agents [202].

There is good evidence that echo contrast agents are valuable in TCD examinations of patients with acute cerebrovascular disease. In an investigation of patients presenting with ischemic strokes and transient ischemic attacks who had insufficient temporal bone windows, 66% of CE-TCDFI studies were conclusive [203]. These findings have been confirmed by a similar study of acute stroke patients in which native transcranial investigations were inadequate [204].

The quality of transtemporal precontrast scans is strongly predictive of the potential diagnostic benefit that is to be expected from application of an intravenous contrast agent. In patients whose intracranial structures are not visible in B-mode imaging and whose vessel segments are not depicted with CDFI, there is little chance that the use of a contrast agent will provide diagnostic confidence [205]. This has also been shown in patients with acute cerebral ischemia. Precontrast identification of any cerebral artery provided an overall accuracy of 97% in predicting a conclusive investigation with contrast agent, while in those without precontrast vessel identification there were no conclusive studies [203].

Vertebral and basilar arteries
Examinations of the intracranial vertebral arteries and the basilar artery are also facilitated with echo contrast agents. Insonation through the foramen magnum when using color-coded duplex sonography and an echo-contrast agent can increase the depth at which vessels can be identified and improve the number of pathologic findings not seen in native scans by about 20% [206]. Moreover, echo-contrast enhancement of the vertebral and basilar arteries may significantly increase diagnostic confidence. As in the examination of the carotid arteries, however, the relative merits of using CE-TCDFI and PDI for assessing the intracranial vertebrobasilar system remain unclear. One study comparing these two modalities concluded that CE-TCDFI and power Doppler sonography are equally effective in visualizing the vertebrobasilar system [207]. Conclusive studies on the role of contrast agents in investigation of the basilar artery are lacking.

Intracranial aneurysms
CE-TCDFI and contrast-enhanced PDI (CE-PDI) employing Levovist have been used to detect and measure the size of intracranial aneurysms [208]. Although CE-PDI missed four of 36 angiographically verified aneurysms, measurements of aneurysm size correlated well with angiographic findings. Other ultrasound studies have suggested that aneurysm dimensions may vary with intracranial pressure (ICP), being larger and less pulsatile at low ICP and smaller but more pulsatile at high ICP [209]. Intraoperative TCDFI allows characterization and localization of aneurysms [210] as well as identification of vessels potentially threatened by clipping [211], whereas intraoperative microvascular Doppler sonography has been shown to be an effective alternative to intraoperative angiography for assessment of vessel patency in aneurysm surgery [212]. An important question remains, whether or not, in cases of acute SAH, transcranial ultrasound is capable of detecting not only the bleeding aneurysm, but also additional asymptomatic aneurysms that may require neurosurgical intervention.

Arteriovenous malformations

Transcranial CE-PDI with Levovist has also been used to evaluate AVM [213]. In one study, CE-PDI identified all angiographically confirmed AVM in patients with adequate temporal bone windows. Although this technique slightly underestimated AVM size, it consistently showed feeding arteries. Coincidental blood supply from another intracranial or extracranial vessel, however, was missed by CE-PDI in all cases. These results are encouraging and demonstrate the potential of CE-PDI for evaluation and follow-up of AVM.

Neurosonology in stroke monitoring

Monitoring of thrombolysis

Recanalization time as determined *in vitro* is an important measure of thrombolysis when the clot is exposed to tissue plasminogen activator (tPA). This is usually given as the time for complete clot dissolution with washout to the distal vasculature and the veins. In human stroke, complete recanalization correlates with clinical recovery as predicted from animal models. Recanalization, however, is a process that often begins many minutes before restoration of cerebral blood flow (CBF), since tPA binding and activity on the clot surface are proportional to the area exposed to blood flow. Once recanalization starts, the clot softens and partially dissolves. This results in an improvement of residual flow that allows more tPA to bind with fibrinogen sites. This process facilitates clot lysis and continually improves residual flow until the clot breaks up under the pressure of arterial blood pulsations.

Recanalization time may be an important clinical parameter of thrombolysis. While prolonged clot dissolution delays complete recanalization and may be associated with a longer duration of cerebral ischemia, a sudden blood flow increase may disrupt the blood–brain barrier and lead to edema or hemorrhage. Alexandrov et al. have recently addressed this issue using real-time ultrasound monitoring of residual flow signals during thrombolysis with tPA in patients with occlusion of the MCA or basilar artery [214]. In their study, recanalization was classified as sudden (abrupt appearance of a normal or stenotic low-resistance signal), stepwise (flow improvement over 1 to 29 minutes), or slow ($\geq$30 minutes). The results showed that recanalization began at a median of 17 minutes and was completed at 35 minutes after tPA bolus, with a mean duration of recanalization of 23 ± 16 minutes. Complete recanalization occurred considerably faster (median 10 minutes) than partial recanalization (median 30 minutes). Importantly, rapid arterial recanalization was associated with better short-term improvement, whereas slow flow improvement and dampened flow signals were less favorable prognostic signs. By providing valuable information on temporal patterns of recanalization, these findings may assist in selection of patients for additional pharmacologic or interventional treatment.

Detection of MES by TCD at the site of arterial obstruction can indicate clot dissolution. Clusters of MES have been detected distal to a high-grade M_1 stenosis preceding spontaneous clinical recovery, and minimal MCA flow signals followed by MES, increased velocities, and normal flow signals have been documented over a period of 2 minutes preceding complete recanalization [215]. Further studies are needed to establish the role of MES detection in monitoring of thrombolytic therapy.

Monitoring of midline shift

Transcranial color-coded sonography is a noninvasive, easily reproducible, and reliable method for monitoring midline dislocation of the third ventricle in stroke patients [216]. It is well suited for monitoring the space-occupying effect of both supra- and infratentorial strokes during treatment on critical care and stroke units [217]. The technique can also be used to facilitate the identification of patients who are unlikely to survive without decompressive craniectomy [218].

Assessment of vasospasm

TCD has become a standard examination procedure for detection, quantification, and follow-up of vasospasms after SAH [94,219,220]. Vasospasms generally occur at the 4th day after SAH, while peak flow velocities can be observed between the 11th and 18th days. Normalization of flow velocities occurs within the 3rd or 4th week after SAH. Rapid increase of velocities 4–8 days following SAH is associated with an increased risk of ischemic stroke.

Although early reports claimed that TCD results mirror the degree of obstruction commonly demonstrated in angiograms of stroke-prone patients after SAH, recent observations have questioned a simple focal narrowing of the arterial lumen, analogous to that in atherosclerotic disease, as the cause of altered Doppler flow patterns following SAH. The pathophysiology of subarachnoid vasospasm is complex. Elevated ICP may lead to an increase in vasomotor resistance of capillary and arteriolar vessels with consequent dampening of the Doppler flow velocity in major proximal arteries. This may result in false-negative Doppler results despite angiographically demonstrable vasospasm. Moreover, local flow turbulence may be found despite a normal appearance of the angiogram if peripheral vasomotor dysregulation and large vessel vasoconstriction occur subsequent to SAH. Importantly, TCD findings in patients with SAH are greatly influenced by changing therapeutic concepts. Only 28% of patients treated with calcium channel blockers have a significant increase in flow velocities prior to the onset of delayed ischemic stroke, suggesting that vasospasm may occur in more distal arterial segments inaccessible to TCD insonation [221]. TCD is further limited in patients with SAH by its relatively poor diagnostic accuracy in the ACA territory, a frequent site of aneurysms [222].

Increased intracranial pressure

TCD can be useful in monitoring ICP in patients with bleeding diatheses and other contraindications to invasive ICP monitoring. Simultaneous recordings of Doppler signals of the basal cerebral arteries, systemic blood pressure, and ICP with epidural devices have shown that a progressive reduction in diastolic and systolic velocities can occur with increasing ICP. Moreover, various patterns of flow alteration have been demonstrated in different regions of the brain, indicating the existence of varying pressure gradients inside the skull [223]. When the ICP rises above that of the diastolic blood pressure, Doppler signals of the basal cerebral arteries are severely altered. Mild or moderate increases in ICP, however, can be compensated for by an increase in the systemic blood pressure, thus resulting in normal TCD findings. Measurements of the absolute ICP value cannot be performed with TCD, but changes in TCD parallel changes in ICP, assuming a constant arterial CO_2 content and a constant degree of distal vasoconstriction. Thus, at least under certain conditions, a quantitative estimation of the ICP could be performed based on consistent relationships between flow velocity parameters recorded from intracranial arteries, and continuous but noninvasive arterial blood pressure measurement. Schmidt et al. supported this concept and showed that a mathematical model could predict ICP modulations from shapes of arterial blood flow and pulse noninvasively [224]. These preliminary findings suggest that TCD may prove useful in evaluating strategies to improve cerebral autoregulation as well as in the optimal management of ICP control.

Functional studies

The introduction of bilateral continuous TCD monitoring has resulted in the development of a variety of new sophisticated applications as supplementary tools to positron emission tomography and functional MRI studies. These include evaluation of functional recovery after stroke.

Recent studies have suggested that changes in cerebral perfusion during motor activity in stroke patients with early recovery of motor function may be monitored by TCD [225,226]. Increased flow velocities in both the contralateral and ipsilateral MCAs during motor tasks have been demonstrated, suggesting that areas of the healthy hemisphere can be activated soon after a focal ischemic injury and contribute to the positive evolution of a functional deficit. This phenomenon of ipsilateral activation is not transient because it is evident months after stroke onset. In patients with Broca aphasia following ischemic stroke, a similar increase

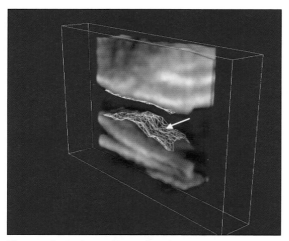

Figure 7. A three-dimensional volume rendering of an atherosclerotic plaque of the internal carotid artery using compounded reconstruction techniques for B-mode imaging. A grid on the plaque surface demonstrates a surface defect (arrow) corresponding to a traumatic plaque rupture.

in MCA flow velocities has been detected after successful speech therapy, providing additional support for contralateral involvement in functional recovery after stroke [227].

New technologies in ultrasonographic stroke imaging

Three-dimensional ultrasound
3-D ultrasound can be used for both qualitative and quantitative analysis of plaques in the carotid artery. Surface features of carotid plaques, not readily appreciated in conventional two-dimensional (2-D) B-mode scanning, can be clearly demonstrated by 3-D ultrasound. In some cases, this may lead to a diagnosis not obtainable with other imaging techniques. This was shown recently in a case of traumatic plaque rupture (see **Figure 7**) occurring during karate training [228]. In a quantitative sense, the volumetric potential of 3-D ultrasound has important clinical implications in serial follow-up studies for observing the progression or regression of stenotic lesions and for evaluating the outcome of interventional procedures such as endarterectomy or stent placement [229]. The assessment of plaque size by B-mode imaging alone has important limitations, including a low interobserver reproducibility. First attempts at volume quantification of carotid plaques were undertaken several years ago and involved tedious manual tracing of sequential B-mode slices [230]. Rapid developments in computer hardware and software then made this task feasible in the clinical setting. The use of an advanced imaging system for acquisition and offline analysis of electrocardiogram-gated, equidistant axial B-mode scans allows a reliable

121. Ries F, Eicke M. Auswirkungen der extrakorporalen Zirkulation auf die intrazerebrale Hämodynamik - Erklärung postoperativer neuropsychiatrischer Komplikationen. In: Widder B, Editor. *Transkranielle Doppler-Sonographie bei zerebrovaskulären Erkrankungen.* Berlin Heidelberg New York: Springer, 1987: 100–3.

122. Bunegin L, Wahl D, Albin MS. Detection and volume estimation of embolic air in the middle cerebral artery using transcranial Doppler sonography. *Stroke* 1994;25(3):593–600.

123. Jansen C, Ramos LM, van Heesewijk JP et al. Impact of microembolism and hemodynamic changes in the brain during carotid endarterectomy. *Stroke* 1994;25(5):992–7.

124. Gaunt ME, Martin PJ, Smith JL et al. Clinical relevance of intraoperative embolization detected by transcranial Doppler ultrasonography during carotid endarterectomy: a prospective study of 100 patients. *Br J Surg* 1994;81(10):1435–9.

125. Siebler M, Sitzer M, Steinmetz H. Detection of intracranial emboli in patients with symptomatic extracranial carotid artery disease. *Stroke* 1993;1992:1652–4.

126. Siebler M, Sitzer M, Rose G et al. Silent cerebral embolism caused by neurologically symptomatic high–grade carotid stenosis. Event rates before and after carotid endarterectomy. *Brain* 1993;116(Pt 5):1005–15.

127. Grosset DG, Georgiadis D, Abdullah I et al. Doppler emboli signals vary according to stroke subtype. *Stroke* 1994;25(2):382–4.

128. Georgiadis D, Grosset DG, Quin RO et al. Detection of intracranial emboli in patients with carotid disease. *Eur J Vasc Surg* 1994;8(3):309–14.

129. Markus HS, Droste DW, Brown MM. Detection of asymptomatic cerebral embolic signals with Doppler ultrasound. *Lancet* 1994;343(8904):1011–2.

130. Grosset DG, Cowburn P, Georgiadis D et al. Ultrasound detection of cerebral emboli in patients with prosthetic heart valves. *J Heart Valve Dis* 1994;3(2):128–32.

131. Georgiadis D, Mallinson A, Grosset DG et al. Coagulation activity and emboli counts in patients with prosthetic cardiac valves. *Stroke* 1994;25(6):1211–4.

132. Diehl RR, Sliwka U, Rautenberg W et al. Evidence for embolization from a posterior cerebral artery thrombus by transcranial Doppler monitoring. *Stroke* 1993;24:606–8.

133. Consensus Committee of the Ninth International Cerebral Hemodynamics Symposium. Basic identification criteria of Doppler microembolic signals. *Stroke* 1995;26(6):1123.

134. Georgiadis D, Baumgartner RW, Karatschai R et al. Further evidence of gaseous embolic material in patients with artificial heart valves. *J Thorac Cardiovasc Surg* 1998;115(4):808–10.

135. Valdueza JM, Harms L, Doepp F et al. Venous microembolic signals detected in patients with cerebral sinus thrombosis. *Stroke* 1997;28(8):1607–9.

136. Georgiadis D, Kaps M, Siebler M et al. Variability of Doppler microembolic signal counts in patients with prosthetic cardiac valves. *Stroke* 1995;26(3):439–43.

137. Markus H, Bland JM, Rose G et al. How good is intercenter agreement in the identification of embolic signals in carotid artery disease? *Stroke* 1996;27(7):1249–52.

138. Van Zuilen EV, Mess WH, Jansen C et al. Automatic embolus detection compared with human experts. A Doppler ultrasound study. *Stroke* 1996;27(10):1840–3.

139. Ringelstein EB, Droste DW, Babikian VL et al. Consensus on microembolus detection by TCD. International Consensus Group on Microembolus Detection. *Stroke* 1998;29(3):725–9.

140. Georgiadis D, Wenzel A, Zerkowski HR et al. Influence of transducer frequency on Doppler microemboli signals in an in vivo model. *Neurol Res* 1998;20(3):198–200.

141. Keunen RW, Stam CJ, Tavy DL et al. Preliminary report of detecting microembolic signals in transcranial Doppler time series with nonlinear forecasting. *Stroke* 1998;29(8):1638–43.

142. Ries F, Tiemann K, Pohl C et al. High-resolution emboli detection and differentiation by characteristic postembolic spectral patterns. *Stroke* 1998;29(3):668–72.

143. Roy E, Abraham P, Montresor S et al. The narrow band hypothesis: an interesting approach for high-intensity transient signals (HITS) detection. *Ultrasound Med Biol* 1998;24(3):375–82.

144. International Workshop on Cerebral Embolism. *Cerebrovasc Dis* 1995;5:67–158.

145. Rautenberg W, Ries S, Bäzner H et al. Emboli detection by TCD monitoring. *Can J Neurol Sci* 1993;20:138–9.

146. Grosset DG, Georgiadis D, Kelman AW et al. Quantification of ultrasound emboli signals in patients with cardiac and carotid disease. *Stroke* 1993;24(12):1922–4.

147. van Zuilen EV, Moll FL, Vermeulen FE et al. Detection of cerebral microemboli by means of transcranial Doppler monitoring before and after carotid endarterectomy. *Stroke* 1995;26(2):210–3.

148. Markus HS, Thomson N, Brown MM. Asymptomatic cerebral embolic signals in symptomatic and asymptomatic carotid artery disease. *Brain* 1995;118:1005–11.

149. Daffertshofer M, Ries S, Schminke U et al. High-intensity transient signals in patients with cerebral ischemia. *Stroke* 1996;27:1844–9.

150. Koennecke HC, Mast H, Trocio SHJ et al. Frequency and determinants of microembolic signals on transcranial Doppler in unselected patients with acute carotid territory ischemia. A prospective study. *Cerebrovasc Dis* 1998;8(2):107–12.

151. Sliwka U, Lingnau A, Stohlmann WD et al. Prevalence and time course of microembolic signals in patients with acute stroke; a prospective study. *Stroke* 1997;28:358–63.

152. Tong DC, Albers GW. Transcranial Doppler-detected microemboli in patients with acute stroke. *Stroke* 1995;26(9):1588–92.

153. Forteza AM, Babikian VL, Hyde C et al. Effect of time and cerebrovascular symptoms on the prevalence of microembolic signals in patients with cervical carotid stenosis. *Stroke* 1996;27:687–90.

154. Wijman CA, Babikian VL, Matjucha IC et al. Cerebral microembolism in patients with retinal ischemia. *Stroke* 1998;29(6):1139–43.

155. Eicke BM, von Lorentz J, Paulus W. Embolus detection in different degrees of carotid disease. *Neurol Res* 1995;17(3):181–4.

156. Sitzer M, Muller W, Siebler M et al. Plaque ulceration and lumen thrombus are the main sources of cerebral microemboli in high-grade internal carotid artery stenosis. *Stroke* 1995;26(7):1231–3.

157. Valton L, Larrue V, Arrué P et al. Asymptomatic cerebral embolic signals in patients with carotid stenosis: correlation with appearance of plaque ulceration on angiography. *Stroke* 1995;26(5):813–5.

158. Oliveira V, Batista P, Soares F et al. HITS in internal carotid dissections. *Cerebrovasc Dis* 2001;11(4):330–4.

159. Molina CA, Alvarez-Sabin J, Schonewille W et al. Cerebral microembolism in acute spontaneous internal carotid artery dissection. *Neurology* 2000;55(11):1738–40.

160. Schauble B, Wijman CA, Koleini B et al. Ophthalmic artery microembolism in giant cell arteritis. *J Neuroophthalmol* 2000;20(4):273–5.

161. Fukuchi K, Kusuoka H, Watanabe Y et al. Correlation of sequential MR images of microsphere-induced cerebral ischemia with histologic changes in rats. *Invest Radiol* 1999;34(11):698–703.

162. Behrens S, Daffertshofer M, Hennerici MG. Stroke treatment guided by transcranial Doppler monitoring in a patient unresponsive to standard regimens. *Cerebrovasc Dis* 1999;9(3):175–7.

163. Siebler M, Kleinschmidt A, Sitzer M et al. Cerebral microembolism in symptomatic and asymptomatic high-grade internal carotid artery stenosis. *Neurology* 1994;44(4):615–8.

164. Babikian VL, Hyde C, Pochay V et al. Clinical correlates of high-intensity transient signals detected on transcranial Doppler sonography in patients with cerebrovascular disease. *Stroke* 1994;25(8):1570–3.

165. Valton L, Larrue V, le Traon AP et al. Microembolic signals and risk of early recurrence in patients with stroke or transient ischemic attack. *Stroke* 1998;29(10):2125–8.

166. Babikian VL, Wijman CA, Hyde C et al. Cerebral microembolism and early recurrent cerebral or retinal ischemic events. *Stroke* 1997;28(7):1314–8.

167. Hennerici M. High intensity transcranial signals (HITS): a questionable "Jackpot" for the prediction of stroke risk. *J Heart Valve Dis* 1994;3:124–5.

168. Ringelstein EB, Droste DW, Babikian VL et al. Consensus on microembolus detection by TCD. International Consensus Group on Microembolus Detection. *Stroke* 1998;29(3):725–9.

169. Valdueza JM, Schmierer K, Mehraein S et al. Assessment of normal flow velocity in basal cerebral veins. A transcranial doppler ultrasound study. *Stroke* 1996;27(7):1221–5.

170. Baumgartner RW, Gonner F, Arnold M et al. Transtemporal power- and frequency-based color-coded duplex sonography of cerebral veins and sinuses. *AJNR Am J Neuroradiol* 1997;18(9):1771–81.

171. Stolz E, Kaps M, Kern A et al. Transcranial color-coded duplex sonography of intracranial veins and sinuses in adults. Reference data from 130 volunteers. *Stroke* 1999;30(5):1070–5.

172. Valdueza JM, Hoffmann O, Weih M et al. Monitoring of venous hemodynamics in patients with cerebral venous thrombosis by transcranial Doppler ultrasound. *Arch Neurol* 1999;56(2):229–34.

173. Canhao P, Batista P, Ferro JM. Venous transcranial Doppler in acute dural sinus thrombosis. *J Neurol* 1998;245(5):276–9.

174. Stolz E, Kaps M, Dorndorf W. Assessment of intracranial venous hemodynamics in normal individuals and patients with cerebral venous thrombosis. *Stroke* 1999;30(1):70–5.

175. Ries S, Steinke W, Neff KW et al. Echocontrast-enhanced transcranial color-coded sonography for the diagnosis of transverse sinus venous thrombosis. *Stroke* 1997;28(4):696–700.

176. Schwartz A, Rautenberg W, Hennerici M. Dolichoectatic intracranial arteries: review of selected aspects. *Cerebrovasc Dis* 1993;3:273–9.

177. Rautenberg W, Aulich A, Röther J et al. Stroke and dolichoectatic intracranial arteries. *Neurol Res* 1992;14:201–3.

178. Adams RJ, Nichols FT, Aaslid R et al. Cerebral vessel stenosis in sickle cell disease: criteria for detection by transcranial Doppler. *Am J Pediatr Hematol Oncol* 1990;12(3):277–82.

179. Adams RJ, Nichols FT, Figueroa R et al. Transcranial Doppler correlation with cerebral angiography in sickle cell disease. *Stroke* 1992;23(8):1073–7.

180. Bogousslavsky J, Despland PA, Regli F et al. Postpartum cerebral angiopathy: reversible vasoconstriction assessed by transcranial Doppler ultrasounds. *Eur Neurol* 1989;29(2):102–5.

181. Chimowitz MI, Nemec JJ, Marwick TH et al. Transcranial Doppler ultrasound identifies patients with right-to-left cardiac or pulmonary shunts. *Neurology* 1991;41(12):1902–4.

182. Di Tullio M, Sacco RL, Venketasubramanian N et al. Comparison of diagnostic techniques for the detection of a patent foramen ovale in stroke patients. *Stroke* 1993;(24):1020–4.

183. Itoh T, Matsumoto M, Handa N et al. Paradoxical embolism as a cause of ischemic stroke of uncertain etiology. A transcranial Doppler sonographic study. *Stroke* 1994;25(4):771–5.

184. Jauss M, Kaps M, Keberle M et al. A comparison of transesophageal echocardiography and transcranial Doppler sonography with contrast medium for detection of patent foramen ovale. *Stroke* 1994;25(6):1265–7.

185. Hamann GF, Schatzer KD, Frohlig G et al. Femoral injection of echo contrast medium may increase the sensitivity of testing for a patent foramen ovale. *Neurology* 1998;50(5):1423–8.

186. Schwarze JJ, Sander D, Kukla C et al. Methodological parameters influence the detection of right-to-left shunts by contrast transcranial Doppler ultrasonography. *Stroke* 1999; 30(6):1234–9.

187. Ophir J, Parker KJ. Contrast agents in diagnostic ultrasound. *Ultrasound Med Biol* 1989;15:319–33.

188. Burns PN. Overview of echo-enhanced vascular ultrasound imaging for clinical diagnosis in neurosonology. *J Neuroimaging* 1997;7(Suppl. 1):S2–14.

189. Van Liew HD, Burkard ME. Bubbles in circulating blood: stabilization and simulations of cyclic changes of size and content. *J Appl Physiol* 1995;79:1379–85.

190. Kabalnov A, Bradley J, Flaim S et al. Dissolution of multicomponent microbubbles in the bloodstream: 2. Experiment. *Ultrasound Med Biol* 1998;24(5):751–60.

191. Chang PH, Shung KK, Levene HB. Quantitative measurements of second harmonic Doppler using ultrasound contrast agents. *Ultrasound Med Biol* 1996;22(9):1205–14.

192. Strandness DE, Eikelboom BC. Carotid artery stenosis–where do we go from here? *Eur J Ultrasound* 1998;7(Suppl. 3):S17–26.

193. Sitzer M, Furst G, Siebler M et al. Usefulness of an intravenous contrast medium in the characterization of high-grade internal carotid stenosis with color Doppler-assisted duplex imaging. *Stroke* 1994;25(2):385–9.

194. Sitzer M, Rose G, Furst G et al. Characteristics and clinical value of an intravenous echo-enhancement agent in evaluation of high-grade internal carotid stenosis. *J Neuroimaging* 1997;7(Suppl. 1):S22–5.

195. Furst G, Saleh A, Wenserski F et al. Reliability and validity of noninvasive imaging of internal carotid artery pseudo-occlusion. *Stroke* 1999;30(7):1444–9.

196. Ries F, Honisch C, Lambertz M et al. A transpulmonary contrast medium enhances the transcranial Doppler signal in humans. *Stroke* 1993;24(12):1903–9.

197. Haggag KJ, Russell D, Brucher R et al. Contrast enhanced pulsed Doppler and colour-coded Duplex studies of the cranial vasculature. *Eur J Neurol* 1999;6(4):443–8.

198. Otis S, Rush M, Boyajian R. Contrast-enhanced transcranial imaging. Results of an American phase-two study. *Stroke* 1995;26(2):203–9.

199. Gerriets T, Seidel G, Fiss I et al. Contrast-enhanced transcranial color-coded duplex sonography: efficiency and validity. *Neurology* 1999;52(6):1133–7.

200. Murphy KJ, Bude RO, Dickinson LD et al. Use of intravenous contrast material in transcranial sonography. *Acad Radiol* 1997;4(8):577–82.

201. Stolz E, Kaps M, Kern A et al. Frontal bone windows for transcranial color-coded duplex sonography. *Stroke* 1999;30(4):814–20.

202. Delcker A, Turowski B. Diagnostic value of three-dimensional transcranial contrast duplex sonography. *J Neuroimaging* 1997;7(3):139–44.

203. Baumgartner RW, Arnold M, Gonner F et al. Contrast-enhanced transcranial color-coded duplex sonography in ischemic cerebrovascular disease. *Stroke* 1997;28(12):2473–8.

204. Nabavi DG, Droste DW, Kemeny V et al. Potential and limitations of echocontrast-enhanced ultrasonography in acute stroke patients: a pilot study. *Stroke* 1998;29(5):949–54.

205. Nabavi DG, Droste DW, Schulte-Altedorneburg G et al. Diagnostic benefit of echocontrast enhancement for the insufficient transtemporal bone window. *J Neuroimaging* 1999;9(2):102–7.

206. Droste DW, Nabavi DG, Kemeny V et al. Echocontrast enhanced transcranial colour-coded duplex offers improved visualization of the vertebrobasilar system. *Acta Neurol Scand* 1998;98(3):193–9.

207. Postert T, Meves S, Bornke C et al. Power Doppler compared to color-coded duplex sonography in the assessment of the basal cerebral circulation. *J Neuroimaging* 1997;7(4):221–6.

208. Griewing B, Motsch L, Piek J et al. Transcranial power mode Doppler duplex sonography of intracranial aneurysms. *J Neuroimaging* 1998;8(3):155–8.

209. Wardlaw JM, Cannon J, Statham PF et al. Does the size of intracranial aneurysms change with intracranial pressure? Observations based on color "power" transcranial Doppler ultrasound. *J Neurosurg* 1998;88(5):846–50.

210. Woydt M, Greiner K, Perez J et al. Intraoperative color duplex sonography of basal arteries during aneurysm surgery. *J Neuroimaging* 1997;7(4):203–7.

211. Mursch K, Schaake T, Markakis E. Using transcranial duplex sonography for monitoring vessel patency during surgery for intracranial aneurysms. *J Neuroimaging* 1997;7(3):164–70.

212. Bailes JE, Tantuwaya LS, Fukushima T et al. Intraoperative microvascular Doppler sonography in aneurysm surgery. *Neurosurgery* 1997;40(5):965–70.

213. Uggowitzer MM, Kugler C, Riccabona M et al. Cerebral arteriovenous malformations: diagnostic value of echo-enhanced transcranial Doppler sonography compared with angiography. *Am J Neuroradiol* 1999;20(1):101–6.

214. Alexandrov AV, Burgin WS, Demchuk AM et al. Speed of intracranial clot lysis with intravenous tissue plasminogen activator therapy: sonographic classification and short–term improvement. *Circulation* 2001;103(24):2897–902.

215. Alexandrov AV, Demchuk AM, Felberg RA et al. Intracranial clot dissolution is associated with embolic signals on transcranial Doppler. *J Neuroimaging* 2000;10(1):27–32.

216. Stolz E, Gerriets T, Fiss I et al. Comparison of transcranial color-coded duplex sonography and cranial CT measurements for determining third ventricle midline shift in space-occupying stroke. *AJNR Am J Neuroradiol* 1999;20(8):1567–71.

217. Bertram M, Khoja W, Ringleb P et al. Transcranial colour-coded sonography for the bedside evaluation of mass effect after stroke. *Eur J Neurol* 2000;7(6):639–46.

218. Gerriets T, Stolz E, Konig S et al. Sonographic monitoring of midline shift in space-occupying stroke: an early outcome predictor. *Stroke* 2001;32(2):442–7.

219. Aaslid R, Huber P, Nornes H. Evaluation of cerebrovascular spasm with transcranial Doppler ultrasound. *J Neurosurg* 1984;60:37–41.

220. Seiler RW, Grolimund P, Aaslid R et al. Cerebral vasospasm evaluated by transcranial ultrasound correlated with clinical grade and CT-visualized subarachnoid hemorrhage. *J Neurosurg* 1986;64:594–600.

221. Laumer R, Steinmeier R, Gönner R et al. Cerebral hemodynamics in subarachnoid hemorrhage evaluated by transcranial Doppler sonography. *Neurosurgery* 1993;31:1–9.

222. Lennihan L, Petty GW, Fink E et al. Transcranial Doppler detection of anterior cerebral vasospasm. *J Neurol Neurosurg Psychiatry* 1993;56:906–9.

223. Hassler W, Steinmetz H, Gawlowski J. Transcranial Doppler ultrasonography in raised intracranial pressure and in intracranial circulatory arrest. *J Neurosurg* 1988;68(5):745–51.

224. Schmidt B, Klingelhofer J, Schwarze JJ et al. Noninvasive prediction of intracranial pressure curves using transcranial Doppler ultrasonography and blood pressure curves. *Stroke* 1997;28(12):2465–72.

225. Silvestrini M, Cupini LM, Placidi F et al. Bilateral hemispheric activation in the early recovery of motor function after stroke. *Stroke* 1998;29(7):1305–10.

226. Caramia MD, Palmieri MG, Giacomini P et al. Ipsilateral activation of the unaffected motor cortex in patients with hemiparetic stroke. *Clin Neurophysiol* 2000;111(11):1990–6.

227. Silvestrini M, Troisi E, Matteis M et al. Correlations of flow velocity changes during mental activity and recovery from aphasia in ischemic stroke. *Neurology* 1998;50(1):191–5.

228. Meairs S, Timpe L, Beyer J et al. Acute aphasia and hemiplegia during karate training. *Lancet* 2000;356:40.

229. Yao J, van Sambeek MR, Dall'Agata A et al. Three-dimensional ultrasound study of carotid arteries before and after endarterectomy;analysis of stenotic lesions and surgical impact on the vessel. *Stroke* 1998;29(10):2026–31.

230. Steinke W, Hennerici M. Three-dimensional ultrasound imaging of carotid artery plaques. *J Cardiovasc Technology* 1989;8:15–22.

231. Delcker A, Diener HC. Quantification of atherosclerotic plaques in carotid arteries by three-dimensional ultrasound. *Br J Radiol* 1994;67(799):672–8.

232. Palombo C, Kozakova M, Morizzo C et al. Ultrafast three-dimensional ultrasound: application to carotid artery imaging. *Stroke* 1998;29(8):1631–7.

233. Griewing B, Schminke U, Morgenstern C et al. Three-dimensional ultrasound angiography (power mode) for the quantification of carotid artery atherosclerosis. *J Neuroimaging* 1997;7(1):40–5.

234. Postert T, Braun B, Pfundtner N et al. Echo contrast-enhanced three-dimensional power Doppler of intracranial arteries. *Ultrasound Med Biol* 1998;24(7):953–62.

235. Deverson S, Evans DH, Bouch DC. The effects of temporal bone on transcranial Doppler ultrasound beam shape. *Ultrasound Med Biol* 2000;26(2):239–44.

236. Klotzsch C, Bozzato A, Lammers G et al. Three-dimensional transcranial color-coded sonography of cerebral aneurysms. *Stroke* 1999;30(11):2285–90.

237. Detmer PR, Bashein G, Hodges T et al. 3-D ultrasonic image feature localization based on magnetic scanhead tracking: in vitro calibration and validation. *Ultrasound Med Biol* 1994;20(9):923–36.

238. Hodges TC, Detmer PR, Burns DH et al. Ultrasonic three-dimensional reconstruction: in vitro and in vivo volume and area measurement. *Ultrasound Med Biol* 1994;20(8):719–29.

239. Leotta DF, Detmer PR, Martin RW. Performance of a miniature magnetic position sensor for three-dimensional ultrasound imaging. *Ultrasound Med Biol* 1997;23(4):597–609.

240. Barry CD, Allott CP, John NW et al. Three-dimensional freehand ultrasound: image reconstruction and volume analysis. *Ultrasound Med Biol* 1997;23(8):1209–24.

241. Meairs S, Beyer J, Hennerici M. Reconstruction and visualization of irregularly sampled three- and four-dimensional ultrasound data for cerebrovascular applications. *Ultrasound Med Biol* 2000;26(2):263–72.

242. Meairs S, Hennerici M. Four-dimensional ultrasonographic characterization of plaque surface motion in patients with symptomatic and asymptomatic carotid artery stenosis. *Stroke* 1999;30(9):1807–13.

243. Porter TR, Xie F, Kricsfeld D et al. Improved myocardial contrast with second harmonic transient ultrasound response imaging in humans using intravenous perfluorocarbon-exposed sonicated dextrose albumin. *J Am Coll Cardiol* 1996;27(6):1497–501.

244. Linka AZ, Sklenar J, Wei K et al. Assessment of transmural distribution of myocardial perfusion with contrast echocardiography. *Circulation* 1998;98(18):1912–20.

245. Postert T, Federlein J, Rose J et al. Ultrasonic assessment of physiological echo-contrast agent distribution in brain parenchyma with transient response second harmonic imaging. *J Neuroimaging* 2001;11(1):18–24.

246. Postert T, Hoppe P, Federlein J et al. Ultrasonic assessment of brain perfusion. *Stroke* 2000;31(6):1460–2.

247. Postert T, Muhs A, Meves S et al. Transient response harmonic imaging: an ultrasound technique related to brain perfusion. *Stroke* 1998;29(9):1901–7.

248. Wiesmann M, Seidel G. Ultrasound perfusion imaging of the human brain. *Stroke* 2000;31(10):2421–5.

249. Seidel G, Algermissen C, Christoph A et al. Harmonic imaging of the human brain. Visualization of brain perfusion with ultrasound. *Stroke* 2000;31(1):151–4.

250. Seidel G, Greis C, Sonne J et al. Harmonic grey scale imaging of the human brain. *J Neuroimaging* 1999;9(3):171–4.

251. Federlein J, Postert T, Meves S et al. Ultrasonic evaluation of pathological brain perfusion in acute stroke using second harmonic imaging. *J Neurol Neurosurg Psychiatry* 2000;69(5):616–22.

252. Postert T, Hoppe P, Federlein J et al. Contrast agent specific imaging modes for the ultrasonic assessment of parenchymal cerebral echo contrast enhancement. *J Cereb Blood Flow Metab* 2000;20(12):1709–16.

253. Uhlendorf V, Hoffmann C. Nonlinear acoustical response of coated microbubbles in diagnostic ultrasound. *Ultrasonics Symp Proc* 1994;1559–62.

254. Goldberg BB, Merton DA, Liu JB et al. Evaluation of bleeding sites with a tissue-specific sonographic contrast agent. *J Ultrasound Med* 1998;17:609–16.

255. Moriyasu F, Kono Y, Kamiyama N et al. Flash echo imaging of liver tumors using ultrasound contrast agent and intermittent color Doppler scanning. *J Ultrasound Med* 1998;17:S63.

256. Forsberg F, Goldberg BB, Liu JB et al. Tissue-specific US contrast agent for evaluation of hepatic and splenic parenchyma. *Radiology* 1999;210(1):125–32.

257. Postert T, Muhs A, Meves S et al. Transient response harmonic imaging: an ultrasound technique related to brain perfusion. *Stroke* 1998;29(9):1901–7.

258. Wei K, Jayaweera AR, Firoozan S et al. Quantification of myocardial blood flow with ultrasound–induced destruction of microbubbles administered as a constant venous infusion. *Circulation* 1998;97(5):473–83.

259. Vincent MA, Dawson D, Clark AD et al. Skeletal muscle microvascular recruitment by physiological hyperinsulinemia precedes increases in total blood flow. *Diabetes* 2002;51(1):42–8.

260. Wei K, Le E, Bin JP et al. Quantification of renal blood flow with contrast-enhanced ultrasound. *J Am Coll Cardiol* 2001;37(4):1135–40.

261. Seidel G, Claassen L, Meyer K et al. Evaluation of blood flow in the cerebral microcirculation: analysis of the refill kinetics during ultrasound contrast agent infusion. *Ultrasound Med Biol* 2001;27(8):1059–64.

262. Rim SJ, Leong-Poi H, Lindner JR et al. Quantification of cerebral perfusion with "Real-Time" contrast-enhanced ultrasound. *Circulation* 2001;104(21):2582–7.

6

Intracerebral hemorrhage

Michael G. Hennerici

Epidemiology and classification

Intracerebral hemorrhage (ICH) accounts for 10%–15% of all cases of stroke and has a high mortality rate, with only one third of affected patients surviving the first year after stroke [1]. Each year, approximately 20/100 000 people suffer an ICH [2], a rate which is expected to increase dramatically during the next 50 years as a result of the increasing age of the population in developed countries.

Depending on the mechanisms underlying brain bleeding, an ICH can be classified as either primary or secondary – the latter is only briefly dealt with in this chapter as this is a special condition associated with bleeding complications from intracranial aneurysms, arteriovenous malformations, or head trauma.

Primary hemorrhage in hypertension and cerebral amyloid angiopathy

Primary ICH often originates from spontaneous rupture of microaneurysms caused by small vessel disease in the presence of chronic hypertension [3–5]. It often affects deep brain structures involved in ischemic microangiopathy, e.g., midline structures such as the basal ganglia, brainstem, and cerebellum (see **Figure 1**). It is therefore often called 'deep brain' hemorrhage.

Another category of primary ICH, 'lobar' ICH, has been described in a group of elderly patients; it affects frontal, parietal, temporal, or occipital, subcortical and cortical structures in the absence of hypertension [6]. Pathogenetically, it is often caused by amyloid deposition in the intracranial vasculature. Amyloid is a homogeneous eosinophilic β-protein found in the neuronal tissue and small vessels of persons usually >60 years of age, and is sometimes associated with antecedent memory loss, which is characteristic in patients developing Alzheimer's disease.

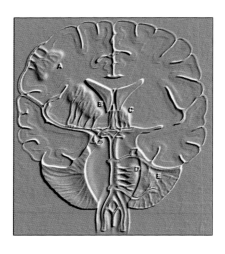

Figure 1. Schematic drawing of preferential sites of both ischemic and hemorrhagic lesions in deep midline structures associated with hypertension such as the basal ganglia, brainstem, and cerebellum, but also subcortical territories of small perforating arteries (modified from Qureshi et al. [53]).

Risk factors

Age

The incidence of both hypertension and cerebral amyloid deposition increases with age, which is the most important risk factor. In the Northern-Manhattan Stroke Study, the annual incidence of lobar ICH was 8–10 cases per 100 000 patients and accounted for one third of all cases of ICH in nontraumatic circumstances [2].

Hypertension

Hypertension is the most important treatable risk factor in all stroke patients. Antihypertensive medication reduces the incidence of not only ischemic stroke but also ICH [7].

Alcohol

Excessive use of alcohol further increases the risk of ICH, mainly by impairing blood coagulation [8,9].

High serum cholesterol levels

Other risk factors of less established significance include high serum cholesterol levels, especially in patients with the $\epsilon2$ or $\epsilon4$ alleles of the apolipoprotein E gene. These alleles are reported to increase the risk of recurrent hemorrhage by 3–5 times in patients with lobar ICH related to amyloid angiopathy [10].

Low serum cholesterol levels

Conversely, recent prospective studies have shown that hemorrhagic stroke occurs more frequently in individuals with low serum cholesterol [11–13]; consequently, lipid-lowering treatment might increase the risk of hemorrhagic stroke [14].

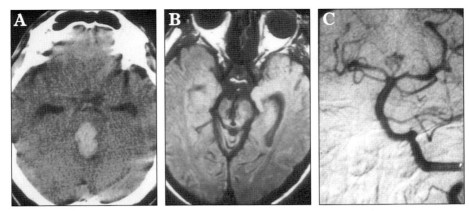

Figure 2. Secondary intracerebral hemorrhage in a patient with arteriovenous malformation in the upper brainstem arising from the basilar artery (A: computed tomography image; B: magnetic resonance imaging scan; and C: angiogram).

However, a recent report of a cohort of 114 793 men, followed over 6 years, showed that low serum cholesterol levels are not an independent risk factor for ICH or subarachnoid hemorrhage (SAH) [15]. This may be because the comparatively small number of hemorrhagic strokes in earlier studies might have contributed to an underestimation of this type of stroke, together with former less conclusive use of brain imaging technologies to separate hemorrhagic from ischemic stroke.

Vascular abnormalities

Secondary ICH occurs in a small number of patients with vascular abnormalities, such as arteriovenous malformations (AVMs), aneurysms, tumors, sinus vein thromboses, vasculitis, and disturbed coagulation (including patients treated with anticoagulants for high thromboembolic risk) (see **Figures 2** and **3**).

Anticoagulation

Anticoagulation increases the risk of ICH by 5–10 times, with absolute ranges of 1% per year or more, even if the international normalized ratio (INR) is within the therapeutic range (see *Pathophysiology of hypertension and CAA-related ICH, page 132*). Recent use of lower intensity anticoagulation therapy and more stringent INR monitoring in dedicated anticoagulation clinics, makes such primary and secondary preventive treatment safer, but these improvements are offset by wider use of anticoagulation therapy in an increasing elderly population who are at higher risk of serious bleeding. Antiplatelet therapy with aspirin also increases the risk of ICH, but to a lesser degree and at a smaller efficacy than has been reported with anticoagulation. Mechanisms explaining how antithrombotic therapies increase intracerebral bleeding have not been elucidated [16], but presence of cerebral amyloid angiopathy (CAA) may be a crucial factor.

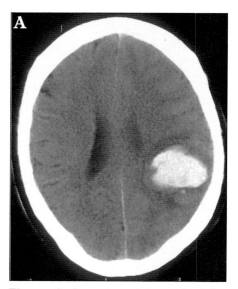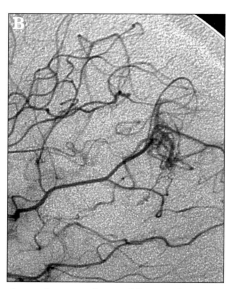

Figure 3. Secondary intracerebral hemorrhage in a patient with arteriovenous malformation in the cortico-subcortical parietal lobe (A: computed tomography image; and B: angiogram).

White matter disease

The presence of white matter disease on computed tomography (CT) and magnetic resonance imaging (MRI) scans is also reported to be an independent predictor of intracerebral bleeding in patients with cerebrovascular disease [17]; a finding that may, more often than previously suspected, reflect the presence of CAA either alone or in coexistence with small vessel disease [18]. Furthermore, asymptomatic microbleeds in gradient echo MRI scans, associated with small vessel disease in some patients – probably coexisting with amyloid angiopathy – may further increase the risk of ICH, especially if a patient is undergoing warfarin treatment for other conditions (see **Figure 4**) [19,20]. Attempts to improve the diagnosis of patients with CAA may also help to better identify patients for warfarin therapy in the presence of risk conditions, such as atrial fibrillation.

In a recent study, Rosand et al. identified an over-representation of patients with warfarin-associated lobar hemorrhage in the presence of the ε2 allele of the apolipoprotein E gene [21]. Although those patients with the ε2 allele represent a small proportion of ICH patients, consideration of such abnormalities in the differential diagnosis of all patients with ICH is necessary in order to utilize the treatment options available, and because of the high risk of hemorrhage recurrence.

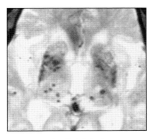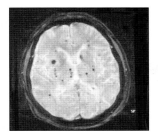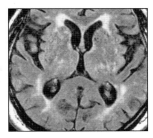

Figure 4. Multiple asymptomatic microbleeds in gradient echo magnetic resonance imaging scans associated with extensive subcortical vascular encephalopathy in hypertensive patients with small artery disease. Predilective sites are the temporal lobes, brainstem, and basal ganglia.

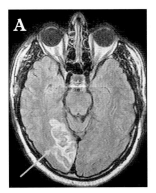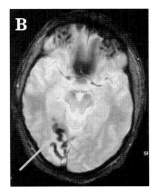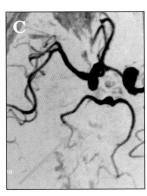

Figure 5. Hemorrhagic infarction (type II) in the posterior cerebral artery territory (A: computed tomography image; B: magnetic resonance imaging scan; and C: angiogram).

Symptomatic hemorrhage secondary to ischemic stroke

Symptomatic hemorrhage secondary to ischemic stroke is defined as clinical deterioration associated with hemorrhagic transformation of any type: hemorrhagic infarction (types I and II) and parenchymal hematoma (types I and II) [22]. According to a *post hoc* analysis of the data set of the European Cooperative Acute Stroke Study II (ECASS II), only parenchymal hematoma type II is associated with an increased risk of clinical deterioration at 24 hours after stroke, while all other types did not increase the risk (see **Figure 5**). Parenchymal hematoma type II has distinct radiologic features, including a dense homogeneous hematoma, >30% of ischemic lesion volume, and significant space occupying effect.

Multiple simultaneous ICH

Multiple simultaneous ICH has only occasionally been studied, and predisposing factors (as well as other physiologic mechanisms) are uncertain. In a recent series including 142 patients with hemorrhagic stroke, only 4 patients demonstrated

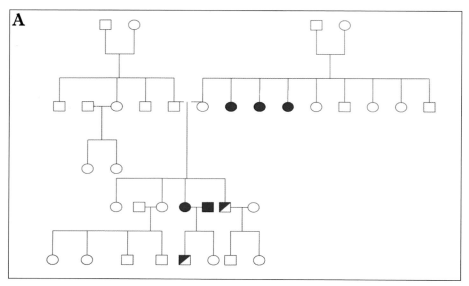

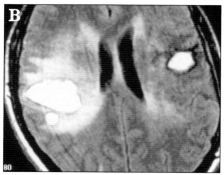

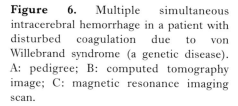

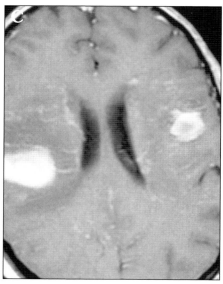

Figure 6. Multiple simultaneous intracerebral hemorrhage in a patient with disturbed coagulation due to von Willebrand syndrome (a genetic disease). A: pedigree; B: computed tomography image; C: magnetic resonance imaging scan.

multiple simultaneous hemorrhages, all of which were due to uncontrolled arterial hypertension. Other mechanisms might include bleeding disorders, vasculitis, hematologic disorders, and anticoagulant therapy, as well as CAA, though sequential hemorrhages are far more common in this condition (see **Figure 6**) [23].

Pathophysiology of hypertension and CAA-related ICH

The majority of deep ICH cases are caused by the rupture of small microaneurysms related to degenerative changes induced by poorly controlled

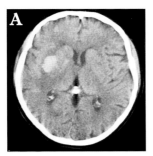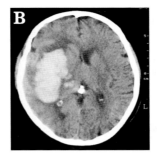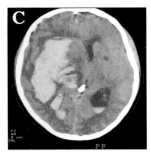

Figure 7. Rapid expansion of intracerebral hemorrhage. The first computed tomography scan (A) was obtained immediately at presentation of the patient in hospital after onset of only mild left-sided hemiparesis. Despite normalization of international normalized ratio values for atrial fibrillation in this anticoagulated patient, a marked clinically asymptomatic expansion of the hematoma was visible within the next 8 hours (B), before severe neurologic deterioration and expansion of the hematoma occurred with ventricular bleeding complications on the computed tomography scan 24 hours later (C).

hypertension. The annual risk of recurrence is 2% if adequate antihypertensive treatment is not provided [24]. Most common signs involve:

- end territories of small cortical branches of the anterior, middle, or posterior cerebral arteries (ACA, MCA, and PCA, respectively)

- ascending lenticulostriate branches of the MCA in the basal ganglia

- thalamogeniculate branches of the PCA in the thalamus

- paramedian branches of the basilar artery in the brain stem

- penetrating branches from the posterior, inferior, anterior inferior, or superior cerebellar arteries in the cerebellum (see **Figure 1**)

Due to their deep location, hematomas extend into the ventricles, and hemorrhage may spread throughout adjacent white matter leaving areas of intact neuronal tissue within the hematoma, forming a potentially substantial portion of salvageable brain tissue in the vicinity of the core of the bleeding (see **Figure 7**). Electron microscopy studies have identified degeneration of the media and smooth muscle cells in the walls of small arterioles as the source of bleeding microaneurysms [3]. The collection of fluid in the region surrounding the hematoma starts the process of neuronal damage, directly as well as indirectly, through disruption of the blood–brain barrier; whereas cerebral ischemia, long believed to result from mechanical compression induced by the hematoma itself, probably plays a less important role [25–30].

Rupture of small and medium sized arteries with deposition of β-amyloid protein forms the basis of lobar CAA-related ICH in the elderly (>70 years of age) in the absence of severe hypertension. They have a lower mortality rate but a greater risk of recurrence than patients with deep cerebral hemorrhage. Occurrence is also associated with the presence of apolipoprotein E ε4 or ε2 alleles. O'Donnell et al. have reported that patients with apolipoprotein E ε4 or ε2 alleles have a relative risk of 3.8% as a predictor of lobar hemorrhage and a 28% risk of recurrence over 2 years for carriers of both or either allele; as compared with 10% for patients with the normal variant, ε3 [10]. The authors also found that prior symptomatic brain hemorrhage was a strong predictor of recurrence, with a 61% risk of recurrence after 2 years. Identification of these genetic markers may be used as a first step in prevention and treatment programs in individual subjects.

Although sporadic cases of CAA-related ICH are suspected to occur more frequently than familial cases, a genetic cause seems likely in both. Different types of amyloid have been described in studies in the Netherlands, Iceland, and Portugal, and some of them have been attributed to autosomal dominant mutations [31,32]. Several forms of genetic disorder associated with ICH and hemorrhagic stroke are listed in **Table 1**.

Unfortunately, a definite diagnosis of ICH related to CAA requires confirmation at autopsy of severe CAA in the presence of lobar hemorrhage with no evidence of any other cause [33,34]. The diagnosis of probable CAA is based on neuropathologic findings in a biopsy specimen of tissue obtained during evacuation of a hematoma or, in the absence of neuropathologic findings, the clinical diagnosis may be based on multiple lobar hemorrhages. Possible diagnosis of CAA is usually documented in patients with a solitary lobar ICH without any other clear cause.

Clinical and imaging investigations

Large brain hematomas usually lead to a rapidly decreasing level of consciousness as a result of increased intracranial pressure (ICP), and direct compression of the midbrain structures in deep ICH [35,36]. Supratentorial ICH (80%) cause contralateral sensorimotor deficits of varying severity and may also present with cortical dysfunction, gaze deviation, aphasia, hemineglect, and hemianopia due to disruption of connecting fibers in the subcortical white matter. Due to the similarity of these signs and symptoms, they cannot be separated from ischemic lesions using pure clinical criteria, but need immediate brain imaging work-up (see **Figure 8**). This is even more of a problem in patients with infratentorial ICH (20%) who may present with the full range of signs indicating brainstem dysfunction with/without involvement of the cerebellum (e.g., supranuclear and

Disorder	Type	Inheritance	Gene/chromosome location
Primary ICH			
ICH			*APOE* gene
CAA			ϵ2 allele
			ϵ4 allele
Hereditary ICH with amyloidosis (Dutch variant)	Monogenic with genetic heterogeneity	AD	Single base mutation (Glu^{693}→Gly) in amyloid beta precursor protein gene on chromosome 21
		AD	Mutation in codon 693 of amyloid precursor protein (APP^{693})
		AD	Mutation in codon 692 of amyloid precursor protein (APP^{692})
Hereditary ICH with amyloidosis (Icelandic variant)	Monogenic	AD	Single nucleotide substitution (Leu^{68}→Gln) in cystatin C gene
Secondary ICH			
IC	Polygenic	AD	
IC1		AD	Chromosome 7q11.2–q21
			Mutations in the gene encoding KRIT1 (Krev-1/rap1a binding protein)
IC2		AD	Chromosome 7p15–13
IC3		AD	Chromosome 3q25, 2–27
Arteriovenous malformations	Polygenic		
HHT (Osler–Weber–Rendu syndrome)			
HHT type 1		AD	Endoglin gene on chromosome 9q
HHT type 2		AD	Activin receptor-like kinase gene on chromosome 12q
Familial venous malformations	Monogenic	AD	Single nucleotide mutation in Tie-2 gene on chromosome 9p
Von Hippel Lindau		AD	Chromosome 3p25–26

AD: autosomal dominant; APOE: apolipoprotein E; CAA: cerebral amyloid angiopathy; HHT: hereditary hemorrhagic telangiectasia; IC: intracerebral cavernous; ICH: intracerebral hemorrhage.

Table 1. Primary and secondary intracerebral hemorrhage resulting from genetic disorders [52].

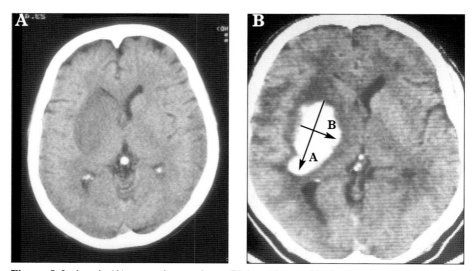

Figure 8. Ischemia (A) versus hemorrhage (B) in patients with similar signs and symptoms only identified by immediate brain imaging studies. A simple method to calculate intracerebral hemorrhage volume is indicated and can be used by estimating the hematoma as half the product of A, B and C, where A is the greatest diameter of the hemorrhage on the computed tomography scan, B the diameter perpendicular to A, and C the number of slices showing hematoma multiplied by the slice thickness (according to [38]).

nuclear oculomotor dysfunctions, unilateral or bilateral sensorimotor deficits, ataxia and nystagmus, dysarthria, fluctuating levels of consciousness, speech and swallowing disturbances, headache, vomiting, vertigo). With increasing ICP, stupor and coma may develop in the initially alert patient within 24 hours of the onset of bleeding, and evacuation of a large hematoma or ventricular puncture may represent life-saving treatment procedures.

A low score on the Glasgow Coma Scale (GCS), a large-volume hematoma, and the presence of ventricular blood on the initial CT scan have been shown to be associated with a very high mortality rate [37–40]: patients who initially had a score of <9 on the GCS and a hematoma volume of >60 mL showed a mortality rate of 90% at 1 month, whereas patients with a score of >9 and a hematoma volume of <30 mL had a mortality rate of only 17% [38]. A rapid method to measure the volume of the hematoma on CT scans is shown in **Figure 8**.

Bleedings from intracranial aneurysms may mimic lobar ICH: in the absence of hypertension the native CT scan may be insufficient and either additional contrast enhancement or MRI/MRA may be required in order to prevent misdiagnosis of aneurysmatic bleedings. This is especially the case if bleedings involve the temporal lobe and the Sylvian fissure, or affect the frontal lobes and basal interhemisphere space where SAH often occur from aneurysms usually originating from the circle of Willis or the large cerebral arteries. In contrast to longstanding belief, MRI, if appropriately performed, is as good as CT, even for the detection of small, acute ICH [41]. Gradient-echo MRI has been used to detect such subclinical hemorrhages, which are visualized because of their hemosiderin deposits (see **Figure 4**). If a definite diagnosis cannot be made, cerebral angiography should be carried out, and lumbar puncture for the analysis of cerebrospinal fluid (CSF) may be useful beyond the confirmation of intracranial bleeding in cases with mycotic aneurysms, or secondary ICH in the presence of focal encephalitis.

In normotensive patients of <45 years, angiography can often detect abnormalities; whereas in hypertensive patients of >45 years, vascular abnormalities are less frequent, especially in cases of deep ICH. In patients with lobar hemorrhage and isolated intraventricular hemorrhage, there may be a need for angiography regardless of age, provided the patient's clinical condition supports this. However, angiography may need to be postponed in some patients until resolution of the hematoma, so as not to miss vascular abnormalities, which are invisible in the acute stage. In contrast, all attempts should be made to avoid misdiagnosis between primary ICH and secondary hemorrhagic transformation of primary ischemia, which is sometimes difficult if a very early brain imaging study has not been performed or if both ischemia and hemorrhage are present simultaneously (see **Figure 9**).

Prognosis and follow-up

For individual prognosis, brain imaging and clinical findings can provide valuable clues: the location and size of the hematoma, the presence of ventricular caps, the likelihood of developing edema, hydrocephalus, and expansion of hematoma often within 24 hours (see **Figure 7**). These findings allow a rapid selection of patients who in light of their GCS score have a good or bad prognosis [42,43]. Follow-up studies using MRI technology can be useful for detecting recurrent – often silent – hemorrhage. Furthermore, CAA may cause diffuse and widespread white matter lesions with/without combined focal hemosiderin deposits [44].

Treatment

The lack of concepts of adequate treatment

While the availability of brain imaging has greatly improved the diagnosis of ICH, morbidity and mortality remain essentially unchanged. No currently utilized therapeutic modalities have been associated with a definitive effect, and long-term outcome data from the few small prospective randomized trials demonstrate the lack of promising treatment concepts. Depending on the physician's and the institution's belief, patients are either treated with aggressive surgical

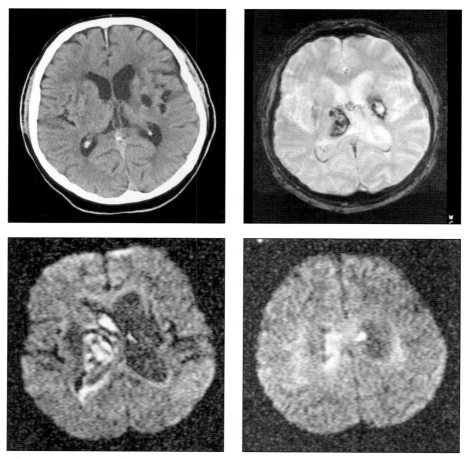

Figure 9. Combination of ischemia and hemorrhage in a patient with previous left lentiform nucleus infarction, due to extensive subcortical small vessel disease and acute onset of signs and symptoms from right deep intracerebral hemorrhage, probably preceded by ischemia as evidenced by a simultaneous small lesion in the left subcortical white matter on diffusion-weighted magnetic resonance imaging.

intervention or conservative monitoring: since neither is evidence-based in the absence of large prospective, randomized, placebo-controlled trials, a first step could be a prospective registry summarizing present strategies and their outcomes.

Conservative management

According to recent observations, immediate intensive/intermediate care, with monitoring of the patient's condition and avoidance of early complications, is useful to minimize poor outcome. Preventive measures include early oxygenation and intubation of stuporous and comatose patients as well as rapid treatment of anticoagulation disturbances if present. Adequate blood pressure, sugar concentration, and fever control with intervention where necessary are also reasonable, as in patients with ischemic stroke. Management is also similar with regards to anticonvulsive treatment: epileptic fits occur in about 20% of patients, more often than in acute ischemia [45]. More invasive monitoring and treatment of ICP is a matter that is under debate; as well as antiedema treatment, sparing corticosteroids in favor of mannitol (mannitol 15%–20%, 125–250 mL, 10–15 minutes). Blood loss due to anticoagulation should be substituted with fresh/frozen plasma and vitamin K; heparin-induced bleedings should be antagonized by protamine sulfate 3 mg/100 IE heparin.

Surgical management
Whether or not surgical removal of the supratentorial ICH is necessary is a question that merits further investigation. Whereas small studies support treatment, at least of medium-sized supratentorial bleedings, functional outcome is probably not better due to early rebleeding or postsurgical excessive edema. Ventricular drainage, a less invasive treatment, mostly failed to show a significant benefit versus conservative monitoring. Only stereotactic puncture, with or without tissue plasminogen activator (tPA) application, seems to have a potential benefit, at least in younger patients with a reasonable GCS score (>8). Patients with small bleedings (<10 mL volume) and GCS scores of >9 usually do well and do not need surgery. According to recent American Heart Association (AHA) consensus statements [46], cerebellar bleedings of >3–4 cm in diameter should be surgically removed; smaller ones should only be removed if signs of ICP develop; however, craniotomy, clot evacuation, or stereotactic tPA administration may be useful in younger patients with moderate supratentorial lobar hemorrhage. Naff et al. [47] published a small study of 20 patients who were given extraventricular drainage and randomized for urokinase versus placebo: admission GCS scores were <8 in 11 patients but ICH volumes were small (mean 6.21 mL). Four patients died within 30 days, which was significantly better than the predicted mortality (86.4%, p<0.00001) for the 20 patients.

The treatment concepts to be studied in clinically based registries or in randomized, multicenter trials [48] should consider patients with poor prognosis (GCS score of <8) with ventricular clots in the midline, or lacking clinical improvement after ventricular drainage; and should be separate from those for patients with a moderate prognosis, younger age, and cerebellar type of ICH. In particular, deep bleedings in midline structures such as the brainstem and thalamus should not be operated on if the underlying bleeding sources (e.g., cavernomas) cannot be removed.

Patients treated for high thromboembolic risks who present with ICH represent a dilemma when considering reinstitution of anticoagulation. The bleeding risk is estimated at 1%–2% per year; however, this is not precisely known because there are very few prospective data available. Since the risk of brain embolism in patients with atrial fibrillation at 1 year may be up to 12% or more, Phan et al. [49] reviewed the short-term management of anticoagulation in 141 patients after ICH. Of the 141 patients in the study, 62 patients died within 30 days of the ICH; 45 of the remaining 79 were given a repeat course of oral coagulation after a median warfarin-free interval of 10 days. The incidence of ischemic stroke at 30 days following warfarin therapy cessation ranged between 3% and 5%; none of those patients who were given repeat anticoagulant therapy had recurrence of ICH during the same period. However, there are contradictory data from smaller more recent series suggesting a higher rate of events during discontinuation of anticoagulation and early rebleedings [50]. A large recent review of the current literature discouraged antithrombotic therapy in patients with any form of recent ICH [51].

Conclusion

Properly conducted clinical trials are required to determine whether or not extension of ICH can be prevented in the first 3–12 hours after bleeding. Ongoing registries and pilot studies will provide useful information to plan such trials appropriately.

References

1. Dennis MS, Burn JP, Sandercock PA et al. Long-term survival after first-ever stroke: the Oxfordshire Community Stroke Project. *Stroke* 1993;24:796–800.

2. Foulkes MA, Wolf PA, Price TR et al. The Stroke Data Bank: design, methods, and baseline characteristics. *Stroke* 1988;19:547–54.

3. Takebayashi S, Kaneko M. Electron microscopic studies of ruptured arteries in hypertensive intracerebral hemorrhage. *Stroke* 1984;14:28–36.

4. Fisher CM. Pathological observations in hypertensive cerebral hemorrhage. *J Neuropathol Exp Neurol* 1971;30:536–50.

5. Cole FM, Yates PO. Pseudo-aneurysms in relationship to massive cerebral hemorrhage. *J Neurol, Neurosurg Psychiatry* 1967;30:61–6.

6. Massaro AR, Sacco RL, Mohr JP et al. Clinical discriminators of lobar and deep hemorrhages. *Neurology* 1991;41:1881–5.

7. Furlan AJ, Whisnant JP, Elveback LR. The decreasing incidence of primary intracerebral hemorrhage: a population study. *Ann Neurol* 1979;5:367–73.

8. Klatsky AL, Armstrong MA, Friedmann GD. Alcohol use and subsequent cerebrovascular disease hospitalisations. *Stroke* 1989;20:741–6.

9. Gorelick PB. Alcohol and stroke. *Stroke* 1987;18:268–71.

10. O'Donnell HC, Rosand J, Knudsen KA et al. Apolipoprotein E genotype and the risk of recurrent lobar intracerebral hemorrhage. *N Engl J Med* 2000;342:240–5.

11. Tanaka H, Ueda Y, Hayashi M. Risk factors for cerebral hemorrhage and cerebral infarction in a Japanese rural community. *Stroke* 1982;13:62–73.

12. Iso H, Jacobs DR Jr., Wentworth D et al. Serum cholesterol levels and six–year mortality from stroke in 350,977 men screened for multiple risk factor intervention trial. *N Engl J Med* 1989;320:904–10.

13. Yano K, Reed DM, MacLean CH. Serum cholesterol and hemorrhagic stroke in the Honolulu Heart Programme. *Stroke* 1989;20:1460–5.

14. Puddey IB. Low serum cholesterol and the risk of cerebral haemorrhage. *Atherosclerosis* 1996;119:1–6.

15. Suh I, Jee SH, Kim HC et al. Low serum cholesterol and haemorrhagic stroke in men: Korea Medical Insurance Corporation Study. *Lancet* 2001;357:922–5.

16. Hart RG, Boop BS, Anderson DC. Oral anticoagulants and intracranial hemorrhage. Facts and hypotheses. *Stroke* 1995;26:1471–7.

17. Gorter JW. Major bleeding during anticoagulation after cerebral ischemia: patterns and risk factors. Stroke Prevention in Reversible Ischemia Trial (SPIRIT). European Atrial Fibrillation Trial (EAFT) study groups. *Neurology* 1999;53:1319–27.

18. Miller JH, Wardlaw JM, Lammie GA. Intracerebral haemorrhage and cerebral amyloid angiopathy: CT features with pathological correlation. *Clin Radiol* 1999;54:422–9.

19. Roob G, Schmidt R, Kapellar P et al. MRI evidence of past cerebral microbleeds in a healthy elderly population. *Neurology* 1999;52:991–4.

20. Greenberg SM, O'Donnell HC, Schaefer PW et al. MRI detection of new hemorrhages: potential marker of progression in cerebral amyloid angiopathy. *Neurology* 1999;53:1135–8.

21. Rosand J, Hylek EM, O'Donnell HC et al. Warfarin-associated hemorrhage and cerebral amyloid angiopathy: a genetic and pathologic study. *Neurology* 2000;10:947–51.

22. Berger C, Fiorelli M, Steiner T et al. Hemorrhagic transformation of ischemic brain tissue: asymptomatic or symptomatic? *Stroke* 2001;32:1330–5.

23. Mauriño J, Saposnik G, Lepera S et al. Multiple simultaneous intracerebral hemorrhages. *Arch Neurol* 2001;58:629–32.

24. Arakawa S, Saku Y, Ibayashi S et al. Blood pressure control and recurrence of hypertensive brain hemorrhage. *Stroke* 1998;29:1806–9.

25. Mul-Bryce S, Kroh FO, White J et al. Brain lactate and pH dissociation in edema: 1H- and 31P-NMR in collagenase-induced hemorrhage in rats. *Am J Physiol* 1993;265:R697–R702.

26. Wagner KR, Xi G, Hau Y et al. Early metabolic alterations in edematous perihematomal brain regions following experimental intracerebral hemorrhage. *J Neurosurg* 1998;88:1058–65.

27. Nath FP, Jenkins A, Mendelow AD et al. Early hemodynamic changes in experimental intracerebral hemorrhage. *J Neurosurg* 1986;65:697–703.

28. Bullock R, Brock-Utne J, van Dellen J et al. Intracerebral hemorrhage in a primate model: effect on regional cerebral blood flow. *Surg Neurol* 1988;29:101–7.

29. Qureshi AI, Wilson DA, Hanley DF et al. Pharmacological reduction of mean arterial pressure does not adversely effect regional cerebral blood flow and intracranial pressure in experimental intracerebral hemorrhage. *Crit Care Med* 1999;27:266–72.

30. Diringer MN, Adams RE, Dunford-Shore JE et al. Cerebral blood flow is symmetrically reduced in patients with intracerebral hemorrhage. *Neurology* 1998;50(Suppl.4):A338.

31. Bornebroek M, Haan J, Maat-Schieman ML et al. Hereditary cerebral hemorrhage with amyloidosis-Dutch type (HCHWA-D): I -a review of clinical, radiologic and genetic aspects. *Brain Pathol* 1996;6:111–4

32. Slooter AJ, Tang MX, van Duijn CM et al. Apolipoprotein ε4 and the risk of dementia with stroke: a population-based investigation. *JAMA* 1997;277:818–21.

33. Greenberg SM, Rebeck GW, Vonsattel JP et al. Apolipoprotein ε4 and cerebral hemorrhage associated with amyloid angiopathy. *Ann Neurol* 1995;38:254–9.

34. Greenberg SM, Vonsattel JP, Segal AZ et al. Association of apolipoprotein ε2 and vasculopathy in cerebral amyloid angiopathy. *Neurology* 1998;50:961–5.

35. Mohr JP, Caplan LR, Melski JW et al. The Harvard Cooperative Stroke Registry: a prospective registry. *Neurology* 1978;28:754–62.

36. Andrews BT, Chiles BW, Olsen WL et al. The effect of intracerebral hematoma location on the risk of brain-stem compression and on clinical outcome. *J Neurosurg* 1988;69:518–22.

37. Qureshi AI, Safdar K, Weil J et al. Predictors of early deterioration and mortality in black Americans with spontaneous intracerebral hemorrhage. *Stroke* 1995;26:1764–7.

38. Broderick JP, Brott TG, Duldner JE et al. Volume of intracerebral hemorrhage: a powerful and easy-to-use predictor of 30-day mortality. *Stroke* 1993;24:987–93.

39. Lisk DR, Pasteur W, Rhoades H et al. Early presentation of hemispheric intracerebral hemorrhage: prediction of outcome and guidelines for treatment allocation. *Neurology* 1994;44:133–9.

40. Tuhrim S, Horowitz DR, Sacher M et al. Validation and comparison of models predicting survival following intracerebral hemorrhage. *Crit Care Med* 1995;23:950–4.

41. Schellinger PD, Fiebach J, Mohr A et al. Stellenwert des Schlaganfall-MRT bei intrazerebralen und subarachnoidalen Blutungen. *Nervenarzt* 2001;72:907–17.

42. Kazui S, Minematsu K, Yamamoto H et al. Enlargement of spontaneous intracerebral hemorrhage: incidence and time course. *Stroke* 1996;27:1783–7.

43. Kazui S, Minematsu K, Yamamoto H et al. Predisposing factors to enlargement of spontaneous intracerebral hematoma. *Stroke* 1997;28:2370–5.

44. Caulo M, Tampieri D, Brassard R et al. Cerebral amyloid angiopathy presenting as nonhemorrhagic diffuse encephalopathy: neuropathologic and neuroradiologic manifestations in one case. *Am J Neuroradiol* 2001;22:1072–6.

45. Pohlmann-Eden B, Hoch DB, Cochius JI et al. Stroke and epilepsy: critical review of the literature. Part I: Epidemiology and risk factors. *Cerebrovasc Dis* 1996;6:332–8.

46. Broderick JP, Adams HP Jr, Barsan W. Guidelines for the management of spontaneous intercerebral hemorrhage: A statement for healthcare professionals from a special writing group of the Stroke Council, American Haert Association. *Stroke* 1999;30(4):905–15.

47. Naff NJ, Carhuapoma JR, Williams MA. Treatment of intraventricular hemorrhage with urokinase: effects on 30-day survival. *Stroke* 2000;31:841–7.

48. Hårdemark HG, Wesslén N, Persson L. Influence of clinical factors, CT findings and early management on outcome in supratentorial intracerebral hemorrhage. *Cerebrovasc Dis* 1999;9:10–21.

49. Phan TG, Koh M, Wijdicks EFM. Safety of discontinuation of anticoagulation in patients with intracranial hemorrhage at high thromboembolic risk. *Arch Neurol* 2000;57:1710–3.

50. Bertram M, Bonsanto M, Hacke W et al. Managing the therapeutic dilemma: patients with spontaneous intracerebral hemorrhage and urgent need for coagulation. *J Neurol* 2000;247:209–14.

51. Keir SL, Wardlaw JM, Sandercock PAG et al. Antithrombotic therapy in patients with any form of intracranial haemorrhage: a systematic review of the available controlled studies. *Cerebrovasc Dis* 2002;14(3–4):197–206.

52. Hademenos GJ, Alberts MJ, Awad I et al. Advances in the genetics of cerebrovascular disease and stroke. *Neurology* 2001;56:997–1008.

53. Qureshi AI, Tuhrim, S, Broderick JP et al. Spontaneous intracerebral hemorrhage. *N Engl J Med* 2001;344:1450–60.

7

Applications of positron emission tomography in ischemic stroke

W-D Heiss

Introduction

Ischemic cell death is a consequence of progressive, deleterious interactions between various circulatory, biochemical, and molecular disturbances [1–5], which, in principle, are amenable to therapeutic intervention. While the many results from biochemical and molecular studies in the laboratory have yet to enter clinical practice, the insight they provide into the dynamics of the development of ischemic damage has had an impact on the management of acute stroke. The severity and extent of permanent neurologic defects are influenced by the amount of tissue suffering impaired blood supply below certain flow thresholds for critical time periods.

Experimental work on ischemic flow thresholds has demonstrated the existence of two critical levels of decreased perfusion. The first is a level representing the flow threshold for reversible neuronal failure (functional threshold). The second is a lower threshold, below which irreversible membrane failure and morphologic damage occur [6]. The range of perfusion values between these limits is termed the 'ischemic penumbra' [7] and is characterized by the potential for functional recovery without morphologic damage, provided that local blood flow can be re-established at a sufficient level and within a certain time window.

Assessment of the pathophysiologic changes leading to ischemic cell damage in a clinical setting is extremely difficult, and most of the biochemical markers cannot be determined in stroke patients. Most clinical examinations do not yield evidence for viability of tissue, and routine studies of the few accessible physiologic variables (by positron emission tomography [PET], single photon emission computed tomography [SPECT], x-ray computed tomography, magnetic resonance imaging [MRI], and magnetic resonance spectroscopy) are limited in most instances by their logistic complexity. Despite these limitations, multitracer PET has obtained the most pertinent results regarding the pathophysiologic changes occurring shortly after ischemic stroke. PET permits the quantitation and three-dimensional (3-D) imaging of distinct physiologic variables [8–10]. This advanced nuclear medicine technology uniquely combines tracer kinetic principles with the specific advantages of coincidence counting and computed tomography (CT), resulting in great methodologic efficiency and flexibility. Depending on the physiochemical properties of the radiotracer on the PET procedure, and on the applied biomathematical model, various major aspects of brain physiology can be investigated at satisfactory spatial and temporal resolution (see **Figure 1**). Therefore, PET appears particularly well suited for studies of the pathophysiologic changes in the course of ischemic stroke.

Methods

Principles of PET

Certain biologically relevant elements, e.g., carbon, nitrogen, oxygen, and fluorine, substituting for a hydrogen atom, have neutron-deficient radioisotopes that decay by emission of positrons (positively charged particles of the mass of an electron). The elements used in PET (termed radionuclides or radiotracers) have very short half-lives of <110 minutes, and, therefore, must be produced close to the PET laboratory, using a low-energy particle accelerator with high beam current, e.g., a cyclotron. Commonly, isotope production is followed by a radiochemical multistep procedure for the synthesis of the final physiologic tracer. The specific advantage of PET over all other nuclear medicine imaging techniques is founded essentially on the principle of coincidence detection. Following emission from the atomic nucleus, the positron takes a path marked by multiple collisions with ambient electrons. Approximately 1–3 mm from its origin, it has lost so much energy that it combines with an electron, resulting in the annihilation of the two oppositely charged particles by the emission at an angle of $180° \pm 0.5°$ of two 511-keV (kilo electron volt) photons that are recorded as coincident events, using pairs of uncollimated (convergent) detectors facing each other. Therefore, the origin of the photons can be localized directly to the straight line between these coincidence detectors.

State of the art PET scanners are equipped with thousands of detectors arranged in up to 24 rings, simultaneously scanning 47 slices of <5 mm thickness. Pseudocolor-coded tomographic images of the radioactivity distribution are then reconstructed from the many projected coincidence counts by a computer, using CT-like algorithms and reliable scatter and attenuation corrections. Typical in-plane resolution (full width at half-maximum) is 5 mm [11]; 3-D data accumulation and reconstruction permits imaging of the brain in any selected plane or view. Spatial resolution and efficiency might be further improved by

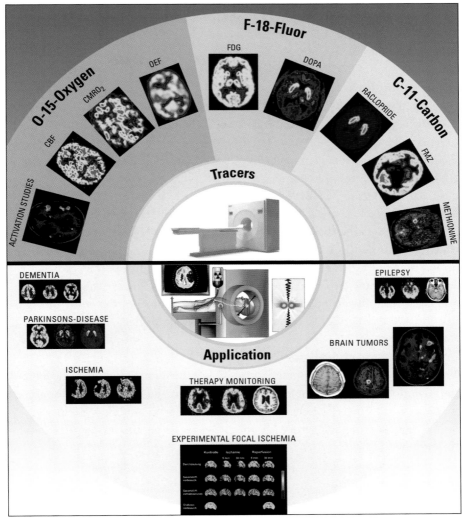

Figure 1. Positron emission tomography: tracers and applications.
CBF: cerebral blood flow; CMRO$_2$: cerebral metabolic rate of oxygen consumption; DOPA:
dihydroxyphenylalanine; FDG: fluoro-2-deoxyglucose; FMZ: flumazenil; OEF: oxygen
extraction fraction.

utilizing a new detector material (e.g., lutetium oxyorthosilicate [LSO]) in the
next generation of PET scanners [12].

Up to the point of data collection and image reconstruction, there is still some
similarity with conventional nuclear medicine imaging techniques: the
radioactivity tomograms represent local tracer concentrations in units of the rate
of nuclear decay that do not have much meaning in physiologic terms.
Only an appropriate biomathematical model describing the compartmental

kinetics of the applied tracer makes it possible to transform these data into images of biological function. Several models require the collection of data by sequential PET scanning for dynamic analysis.

Brain blood flow

Cerebral blood flow (CBF) remains a target of PET studies, despite the fact that the flow is related primarily to brain vascular physiology rather than to neuronal function. This is due to the close coupling of brain blood flow and energy metabolism in physiologic conditions, as well as the procedural and analytical simplicity of CBF measurements. Almost all commonly applied methods for the quantitative imaging of CBF with PET are based on the principle of diffusible tracer exchange. Using ^{15}O-labeled water administered either directly by intravenous bolus injection [13] or by the inhalation of ^{15}O-labeled carbon dioxide, which is converted into water by carbonic anhydrase in the lungs [14], CBF can be estimated from steady-state distributions or from the radioactivity concentration-time curves in arterial plasma and brain. Typical measuring times range between 40 seconds and 2 minutes, and, because of the short biological half-life of the radiotracers, repeat studies can be performed.

Brain energy metabolism

The biochemical energy storage capacity of the brain is extremely limited, and therefore, under physiologic conditions, demand and supply are closely coupled. Furthermore, cerebral energy delivery depends almost exclusively on aerobic glucose metabolism, with the synapse being the major location for consumption [15].

Oxygen consumption

Various PET methods have been developed for determining the cerebral metabolic rate for oxygen (CMRO$_2$), using continuous [14] or single-breath inhalation [16] of air containing trace amounts of ^{15}O-labeled molecular oxygen. All require the concurrent estimation or paired measurement of CBF in order to convert the measured oxygen extraction fractions (OEFs), into images of CMRO$_2$ as given by the product of arterial oxygen concentration, local OEF, and local CBF. Because ^{15}O has a short half-life (123 seconds), an on-site cyclotron is necessary; this and other methodologic complexities limit the use of CMRO$_2$ as a measure of brain function.

Glucose consumption

The cerebral metabolic rate for glucose (CMR$_{glc}$) can be quantified with PET [17,18] using 2-[^{18}F]fluoro-2-deoxyglucose (FDG) and a modification of the three-compartment model equation developed for autoradiography by Sokoloff et al. [19]. Like glucose, FDG is transported across the blood–brain barrier and into brain cells, where it is phosphorylated by hexokinase. However, FDG-6-phosphate cannot be metabolized to its respective fructose-6-phosphate analog, and does not diffuse out of the cells in significant amounts. For this to happen, it must be dephosphorylated again by a phosphatase that is hidden inside the endoplasmic reticulum, and this dephosphorylation is virtually undetectable for approximately 45 minutes. Indeed the distribution of the radioactivity accumulated in the brain remains quite stable between 30–50 minutes after intravenous tracer injection, thus permitting multiple intercalated scans. Using (1) the local radioactivity concentration measured with PET during this steady-state period, (2) the concentration-time course of tracer in arterial plasma, (3) plasma glucose concentration, and (4) a lumped constant (the difference in FDG and native glucose metabolism) correcting for the differing behavior in brain of FDG and glucose, CMR_{glc} can be computed pixel by pixel according to an optimized operational equation [20]. The resulting pseudocolor-coded images reflect all effects on cerebral glucose metabolism, weighted according to the individual, exponentially decreasing FDG plasma concentration-time curve. Because of its robustness with regard to procedure and model assumptions, the FDG method has been employed in many PET studies.

Tracers for neuronal integrity and damage

A simple tracer differentiating between viable and irreversibly damaged tissue is needed for therapeutic decisions, particularly in early stroke. The most reliable procedure – measurement of blood flow and oxygen consumption – is logistically complex and requires arterial blood sampling which is contraindicated if interventional measures, e.g., thrombolysis, are planned. Therefore, several tracers have been investigated as potential markers of neuronal integrity or indicators of hypoxic states.

Central benzodiazepine receptor (BZR) ligands were suggested by Sette et al. as markers for neuronal integrity [21]. They bind to gamma-aminobutyric acid (GABA) receptors, which are abundant in the cerebral cortex and sensitive to ischemic damage. The suitability of central BZR ligands for the detection of early irreversible ischemic damage was tested by comparing defects in binding of a BZR ligand, ^{11}C-flumazenil (FMZ), to defects in energy metabolism and final infarcts after transient middle cerebral artery occlusion in cats [22]. Irrespective of the level of reperfusion, decreases in cortical FMZ binding below ~3.5-times the mean binding in white matter predicted the final infarcts.

Divalent cobalt (Co) isotopes have been suggested as alternative markers of neuronal damage. These ions might visualize changes in neuronal Ca^{2+}

metabolism and increased Ca^{2+} influx into cells, a hallmark in the pathophysiologic cascade of ischemic damage. Studies with $^{55}Co\text{-}Cl_2$ showed accumulation of ^{55}Co primarily in the core and, to a lesser extent, in the periphery of acute and subacute infarcts: accumulation increased over time and was related to the severity of neurologic defects [23].

Markers of hypoxic tissue have also been tested with respect to their capacity to identify penumbral tissue. In animal models of focal ischemia, autoradiography with labeled nitroimidazole derivatives detected increased tracer uptake associated with areas of histologic damage and adjacent areas that appeared intact at follow-up [24]. Only animals with a neurologic deficit showed increased uptake of this tracer. ^{18}F-misonidazole has been used to image cerebral ischemia in man, and an increased uptake was found around the ischemic core, which disappeared in the chronic phase [25,26]. This pattern suggested that 'penumbral' hypoxic tissue had either infarcted or recovered. However, the time course of the tracer kinetics (more than 2 hours between injection and imaging) limits the use of ^{18}F-misonidazole for therapeutic decisions in acute ischemic stroke.

Acute ischemia

The concept of an ischemic penumbra

The term 'ischemic penumbra', originally applied to brain tissue perfused at values between the functional and morphologic thresholds [7], has recently been extended to characterize ischemically affected but still viable tissue with uncertain chances for infarction or recovery [27,28]. Blood flow in penumbral tissue is decreased to the point of causing electrophysiologic silence, and transient, recurrent loss of membrane ion gradients and energy metabolites [29]. In such tissue, flow is insufficient to meet the metabolic demand, but energy metabolism is preserved at a level permitting morphologic preservation of tissue ('misery perfusion') [30]. However, continued ischemic stress and/or additional energy-demanding episodes will exhaust this limited capacity and turn the penumbra into necrotic tissue. Results have accumulated to support the conjecture that a dynamic process of impaired perfusion and unstable energy metabolism is taking place in the ischemic penumbra, and such neighboring tissue inherits the capacity for either recovery or progressive necrosis and growing infarction.

Determination of tissue damage

Assessment of the pathophysiologic mechanisms leading to tissue damage in acute ischemia is of utmost importance for the selection of therapeutic interventions and for the prediction of severity of neurologic deficits. The determination of three critical values is necessary to define the state and the fate of the tissue:

1) the flow threshold for functional impairment – to identify functionally impaired tissue

2) the flow threshold for morphologic damage – to identify irreversibly damaged tissue

3) the time period a tissue tolerates flow decreased to a certain value before it becomes irreversibly damaged – to identify the 'window of opportunity' for recovery of function with reperfusion

These important parameters cannot usually be assessed in acute stages of ischemic stroke in man, and what limits there are regarding ischemic compromise and the chances for recovery have been gleaned from measurements of only a few physiologic variables taken at ill-defined time points after the development of symptoms. Since the changes in physiologic variables that occur in the early hours of ischemia and during reperfusion can only be followed systematically in animal models, the results from experimental focal ischemia are described first. These findings can be used to interpret the observations from multitracer studies in patients with acute stroke.

Experimental studies

Advanced PET equipment has enabled the study of pathophysiologic changes in brain perfusion and metabolism after middle cerebral artery occlusion (MCAO) in baboons [31,32] and cats [33]. The changes in CBF and $CMRO_2$ after MCAO in baboons are moderate, develop with some delay, and are more severe in deep brain structures, whereas in cats, CBF decreases promptly within the whole vascular territory following MCAO. Therefore, the cat MCAO model seems to be better suited to explain the sequence of events after vascular occlusion.

In the cat, changes after MCAO are immediate and severe. Sequential studies of CBF, $CMRO_2$, and CMR_{glc} before, during, and up to 24 hours after MCAO [34] recorded an immediate decrease of CBF within the MCA territory to <30% of control upon arterial occlusion. $CMRO_2$ was less diminished and was preserved at an intermediate level. Consequently, OEF was increased, indicating 'misery perfusion'. This ischemic penumbra spread with time from the center to the borders of the MCA territory. In most instances, the 'misery perfusion' condition was followed by a marked decrease in OEF, reflecting progressive impairment of metabolism and suggesting transition to necrosis spreading from the core to the periphery of the ischemic territory. The infarcts were more or less complete 18–24 hours after MCAO. Occasionally, spontaneous collateral reperfusion resolved the penumbra condition, leading to preservation of the morphologic integrity of the cortex.

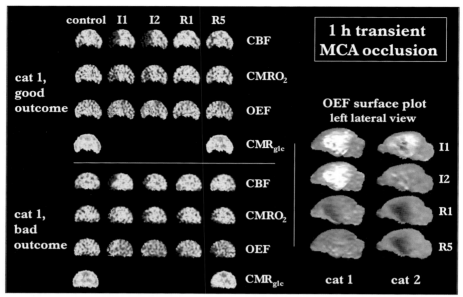

Figure 2. Time course of changes in cerebral blood flow (CBF), cerebral metabolic rate of oxygen consumption (CMRO₂), oxygen extraction fraction (OEF), and the control and late cerebral metabolic rate of glucose (CMR$_{glc}$) in two cats undergoing 1 hour of middle cerebral artery occlusion (MCAO). Cat 1: persistence of increased OEF over the ischemic period indicates viable tissue that can profit from reperfusion. Cat 2: breakdown of oxygen consumption indicates irreversible tissue damage. This tissue cannot benefit from reperfusion. OEF surface plots demonstrate sequential changes during ischemia and reperfusion in the MCA territory with persistence or breakdown of increased oxygen extraction ('misery perfusion') during the ischemic period.
Control: before MCAO; I1: early; I2: late, during MCAO; R1: immediately; R5: 4.5 hours after MCAO.

Reversible MCAO was studied in cats by reopening the MCAO after 30, 60, and 120 minutes [22]. All cats survived 30 minutes of MCAO without developing infarcts. During 60 minutes of MCAO, in animals that survived 24 hours of reperfusion, OEF remained elevated throughout the ischemic episode and this was sufficient to prevent the appearance of large infarcts involving cortical areas (see **Figure 2**). In contrast, the initial OEF increase disappeared during 60 minutes of ischemia in those cats that died during the reperfusion period. Extended postischemic hyperperfusion accompanied large reductions in CMRO₂ and relative CMR$_{glc}$ (rCMR$_{glc}$), large infarcts developed, and intracranial pressure increased fatally. These results highlight the importance of the severity of the ischemia in relation to its duration after reperfusion [35]. A comparison with clinical findings may be justified (see **Figures 2** and **3**). Permanent MCAO resembles the natural course after vascular occlusion, leading to large infarcts in most cases, with a chance of collateral reperfusion that may resolve the 'misery perfusion' and improve outcome. Reopening of the MCA resembles the

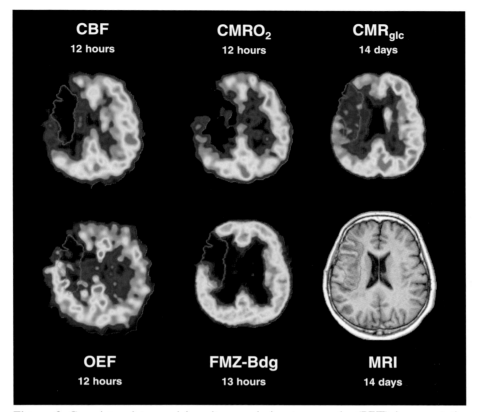

Figure 3. Coregistered transaxial positron emission tomography (PET) images at the caudate/ventricular level of cerebral blood flow (CBF), oxygen extraction fraction (OEF), cerebral metabolic rate of oxygen consumption (CMRO$_2$), steady state flumazenil binding (FMZ-Bdg) at 12 hours, cerebral metabolic rate of glucose (CMR$_{glc}$), and magnetic resonance imaging (MRI) at 2 weeks after moderate left hemiparesis and hemihypesthesia of acute onset in a 52-year-old male patient. The large territorial defect is visible in all PET modalities with different extensions. The contour delineates the cortical infarct as determined on late MRI. FMZ binding precisely predicts the extension of the final infarct, whereas CBF markers delineate a considerably larger volume of disturbed perfusion. In the cortical region outside the infarct with initially disturbed perfusion, OEF is increased, indicating preserved CMRO$_2$ at 12 hours after ictus. The permanently decreased CMR$_{glc}$ in this region could be caused by neuronal loss and/or diaschisis.

(spontaneous) dissolution of vascular occlusion in transient ischemic attack, spontaneous lysis of emboli within the tolerable time period, and therapeutic thrombolysis. In the cat experiments, reperfusion after 30 minutes of MCAO led to a short hyperperfusion period and a fast normalization of flow and metabolism; this may be comparable to a transient ischemic attack. During longer lasting MCAOs, two patterns can be distinguished (see **Figure 2**): a decrease of the OEF during the MCAO reflects fast irreversible damage of tissue, whereas a persistence of elevated OEF indicates preserved viability of tissue over the ischemic period. Forced reperfusion by reopening the MCA cannot salvage irreversibly damaged tissue, but may cause additional damage by inducing edema through leaky vascular endothelium. In such cases, the infarcts are large, and animals die early because of increased intracranial pressure. These courses resemble the deleterious outcome of thrombolytic therapy that is initiated too late, and thus cannot prevent the development of large infarcts, resulting in additional edema and secondary hemorrhagic transformation.

Identification of irreversibly damaged and viable tissue
Human studies

PET studies in patients with acute ischemic stroke have aimed to identify irreversibly damaged and ischemically compromised but viable tissue. In early studies by Kuhl et al. [36], regions with decreased flow and preserved glucose consumption were observed in the first hours after the ictus, and this early mismatch served as an indicator of viable tissue in distinction to other flow-metabolism combinations, e.g., hypoperfusion-hypometabolism, hyperperfusion-hypometabolism, which signaled permanent tissue destruction. Very early in its development, PET with ^{15}O tracers became the gold standard for the evaluation of pathophysiologic changes in early stroke [37]. The quantitative measurement of CBF, $CMRO_2$, OEF, and CBV permitted the independent assessment of perfusion and energy metabolism, and demonstrated the uncoupling of these usually closely related variables.

Early studies, usually comprising a small number of patients, provided data on flow and metabolic values predicting final infarction or suggesting viability at the time of measurement (performed at variable times 5–48 hours after the onset of symptoms). Tissue with an rCBF level of <12 mL/100 g/min, or $rCMRO_2$ (relative $CMRO_2$) <65 μmol/100 g/min, or both, at the time of measurement was usually found to be infarcted on late CT [30,38]. Relatively preserved $CMRO_2$ was accepted as an indicator of maintained neuronal function in regions with severely reduced CBF (see **Figure 3**). This pattern (coined 'misery perfusion' by Baron et al. [39]) served as a definition for the penumbra, which is characterized as the area of increased OEF (up to 80%–100% from the normal value of approximately 40%) [40].

The ischemic penumbra in acute stroke patients

Regions with CBF between 12–22 mL/100 g/min have an unstable metabolic situation. In these areas, infarction will develop if low flow values persist, and they are, therefore, considered to be in the penumbra zone [41]. The upper threshold for the penumbra is also supported by the minimum CBF value determined by PET in regions responsible for transient ischemic attacks [42]. These studies permit the classification of three regions within the disturbed vascular territory:

- the ischemic core usually becomes necrotic when CBF is
  < 12 mL/100 g/min

- the penumbral region has a CBF of between 12–22 mL/100 g/min; tissue in
  this region remains viable, but with uncertain chances for infarction or
  recovery

- the hypoperfused area (CBF is > 22 mL/100 g/min) is not significantly
  damaged by the lack of blood supply

It has to be kept in mind that the classification of tissue changes with time; conversion into infarction and the penumbra is a dynamic process spreading from the core of the ischemic tissue to its border [27,43]. Hence the extent of the penumbra depends on the time of measurement relative to the onset of ischemia: if the penumbra is defined in the first hours of ischemia the volume will be large, and the flow values low (and less than the above mentioned threshold); the volume will be small if it is defined 12–24 hours later. Therefore, in most cases, penumbral tissue characterized by misery perfusion is observed in large tissue compartments within the first hours. In some cases it was detected 16 hours [44], and even up to 48 hours [45], after the onset of stroke. Only a few cases were reported in which misery perfusion persisted chronically [46].

In repeat multitracer PET studies in patients after acute ischemic stroke, it was demonstrated that most tissue compartments showing misery perfusion at the time of the first measurement suffered progressive metabolic derangement and became necrotic over the course of the following 2 weeks [41,45,47]. Only in a few regions, or in special cases, with increased OEF and slightly impaired rCMRO$_2$, was the metabolism preserved close to normal values and did the tissue remain morphologically intact [48,49]. These observations in early stroke prove that penumbral tissue affected by misery perfusion, but with a CMRO$_2$ still greater than the critical threshold, is viable, and may recover if sufficient perfusion is re-established within a critical time window.

Fate of the ischemic penumbra

The identification of flow and metabolic values that are predictive for ultimately infarcted versus noninfarcted penumbral tissue is still a matter of controversy [43]. The values are highly dependent on the separation of cortex from white matter, and suffer from variability and statistical inaccuracy of measurements at low tracer concentrations, but the results of meticulous analyses of PET data collected in a sample of patients studied 7–16 hours after acute stroke [43] are beginning to provide some answers. In the absence of spontaneous

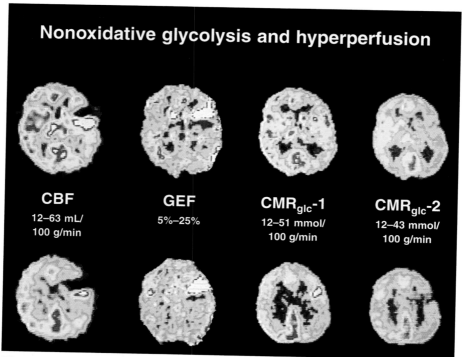

Figure 4. Positron emission tomography (PET) images across the basal ganglia plane (upper row) and the supraventricular plane (lower row) of a patient with partial left middle cerebral artery infarction. Cerebral blood flow (CBF) and cerebral metabolic rate of glucose (CMR$_{glc}$-1) images recorded on the first day after onset of symptoms show a sharply demarcated perfusion deficit and posterior peri-infarct hyperperfusion. Increased glycolysis within the infarct and its surroundings results in an increased glucose extraction fraction (GEF) within the infarct. After 14 days, glucose metabolism is reduced in the infarct and adjacent areas (CMR$_{glc}$-2).

hyperperfusion (see **Figure 4**), a large proportion of the voxels fulfilling the criteria of misery perfusion (CBF of 10–22 mL/100 g/min, CMRO$_2$ greater than the critical threshold of 60 μmol/100 g/min [1.4 mL/100 g/min], OEF >0.7) end up in the final cortical/subcortical infarcts. Spontaneous hyperperfusion is able to prevent structural lesions and leads to excellent clinical recovery [44]. This analysis sets the flow threshold of tissue that might infarct to a maximum of 22 mL/100 g/min. However, some penumbra voxels defined by the same criteria and correlated to the severity of neurologic symptoms at the time of measurement escaped infarction. In these instances, recovery was significantly correlated to the volume of noninfarcted penumbra tissue [49], setting the flow threshold of tissue able to recover to a minimum of 7 mL/100 g/min. These careful analyses indicate that increased OEF is a poor predictor of tissue viability, and that isolated flow measurements at a single time point might be confusing if the pattern over time is not known.

New markers to separate viable from irreversibly damaged tissue
These findings stress the need for a marker of neuronal integrity that can identify irreversibly damaged tissue irrespective of the time elapsed since the vascular attack and irrespective of the variations in blood flow over time. As ^{11}C-FMZ only binds to active GABA receptors, this compound has been used together with [15]O tracers in patients suffering from acute ischemic stroke [50]. The early changes in flow, oxygen consumption, and FMZ binding were compared with permanent disturbances of glucose metabolism and the size of the final infarcts determined on MRI or CT, 12–22 days after the stroke (see **Figure 3**). In all patients, cortical regions with reduced FMZ binding, usually within the larger areas with disturbed blood flow, predicted the final infarcts or, in one case, areas with severely depressed glucose metabolism indicative of marked neuronal loss. The predictive value of reduced FMZ binding was comparable to that of a regional $CMRO_2$ reduction <60 μmol/100 g/min. In these areas, OEF could still be increased, limiting the utility of this variable as an indicator of viability. In contrast to studies with [15]O tracers, the use of the BZR ligand as a marker of neuronal integrity does not necessitate arterial blood sampling, is independent of the cooperation of patients, and has the advantage of superior image quality and the potential of single photon emission computed tomography (SPECT) application. However, studies are restricted to the cortex and require steady state conditions to be reached 30–40 minutes after injection.

By comparing various compartments of reduced flow to the size of the lesion, as established on MRI or CT, 2–3 weeks after the stroke, the impact of the early critical ischemia and of the penumbra on the final infarct can be determined. In an analysis of flow within 3 hours of onset of symptoms in 10 patients [51], critical hypoperfusion below the viability threshold (operationally set to ~12 mL/100 g/min) accounted for the largest portion (70% on average) of the final infarct, whereas penumbral tissue (18%) and initially sufficiently perfused tissue (12%) were responsible for considerably smaller portions of the final infarct.

In another sample of 10 patients studied 2–12 hours after ischemic stroke, determinations of flow and of ^{11}C-FMZ binding in and outside the final infarcts were used to compute cumulative probability curves to predict eventual infarction or noninfarction [52]. Positive and negative prediction limits for CBF (4.8 and 14.1 mL/100 g/min, respectively) and for FMZ binding (3.4- and 5.5-times the mean of white matter, respectively) were determined to define the penumbral range. Using the lower FMZ binding threshold of 3.4-times the mean of white matter for irreversible tissue damage, and the upper CBF value of 14.1 mL/100 g/min for the threshold of critical perfusion at or above which tissue is likely to be preserved, various cortical subcompartments were identified. Of the final cortical infarct (median size, 25.7 cm³) a major portion comprising ~55.1% showed critically decreased FMZ binding, thus predicting necrosis. In ~20.5% of the final infarct, CBF was in the penumbral range (below 14.1 mL/100 g/min) and FMZ binding was above the critical threshold of irreversible damage. Only 12.9% of the final infarct exhibited neuronal integrity and CBF values above the penumbral range.

Therefore, most of the final infarct is already irreversibly damaged at the time of the initial evaluation, several hours after stroke onset. A much smaller portion is still viable but suffers from insufficient blood supply: this tissue may be salvaged by effective reperfusion. An even smaller compartment of viable and sufficiently perfused tissue eventually becomes necrotic, mainly owing to delayed mechanisms: this is the area that may benefit from neuroprotective or other measures targeted at secondary damage. It is clear that early reperfusion is crucial in acute ischemic stroke.

Nonoxidative glycolysis

In acute ischemic infarcts, increased $rCMR_{glc}$ may also be observed up to 14 days after the attack (see **Figure 4**). An indication of increased glycolysis ($rCMR_{glc}$ levels higher than in corresponding gray matter, i.e., above 40 μmol/100 g/min) was present in <10% of over 100 ischemic infarcts studied in our laboratory within the first 4 weeks after onset of symptoms. In recent infarcts, $rCMR_{glc}$ was less reduced than $CMRO_2$ [53], indicating nonoxidative glycolysis. These findings correspond to the detection of lactate in experimental studies and to the results of proton magnetic resonance spectroscopy in human ischemic infarcts [54,55]. Since nonoxidative glycolysis was observed not only during acute ischemia but also under conditions of luxury perfusion [56], it may indicate the presence of anaerobic glycolysis and production of lactate by anaerobic glycolysis as a postischemic metabolic abnormality. In subacute stages, invasion by macrophages contributes to the increase of $rCMR_{glc}$ [57,58].

Chronic deficiencies

Deactivation of remote tissue (diaschisis)

Even the earliest PET studies of ischemic brain lesions [36] revealed reductions of metabolism and blood flow exceeding the extent of morphologically damaged tissue; since then, this has been a regular finding with other functional imaging modalities, such as SPECT. The most conspicuous effect was a reduction of CBF and metabolism in the contralateral cerebellum, called 'crossed cerebellar diaschisis' [59], occurring immediately afterwards and persisting permanently in patients suffering from lesions involving the cortico-pontine-cerebellar pathways [60]. This was obviously due to some neuron-mediated effect, since a primary vascular cause could be excluded on account of the remote vascular territory. Further remote effects included reduction of CBF and metabolism in the ipsilateral cortex (see **Figure 3**) and basal ganglia [61]. Their cause was less clear since selective ischemic neuronal loss [62] or inadequate blood supply could also contribute in these areas. However, similar effects have also been observed in nonischemic lesions, such as brain tumors and intracerebral hematoma, so they seem to be more closely related to the site than to the nature of the primary lesion [63]. Among cortical and subcortical lesions, infarcts of the parietal and frontal lobes most often cause significant reductions of CBF and metabolism in the ipsilateral basal ganglia and the contralateral cerebellum [61,64,65]. This might be explained by damage to cortico-pontine-cerebellar pathways.

Infarcts of the basal ganglia may cause ipsilateral cerebral as well as contralateral cerebellar deactivation. Thalamic infarcts have mainly diffuse ipsilateral cortical effects [66,67], and significant cerebellar deactivation only appears when the internal capsule is involved in the lesion. Infarcts involving the medial thalamic nuclei apparently cause more widespread cortical metabolic reductions (and more nonlocalized symptoms) than those restricted to anterior, ventrolateral, and posterior nuclei [66]. Infarcts of the brain stem and the cerebellum do not usually cause significant asymmetric inactivation of forebrain structures [68].

Remote effects are often the cause of clinical symptoms that are difficult to relate to the actual infarct, and the severity of the metabolic disorder appears to be inversely related to later functional recovery [69]. While several complex neuropsychologic syndromes might be related to inactivation of complex functional networks, e.g., reduced left temporoparietal metabolism in aphasics [70,71], the clinical relevance of the most conspicuous diaschisis – the crossed cerebellar deactivation – is still unclear [68], despite the fact that ataxic hemiparesis and other ataxic syndromes have been noted in single cases secondary to cortical insults [72]. In chronic hemispheric infarcts, neurologic status was related to cerebellar metabolic asymmetry due to the high correlation of cerebellar diaschisis with infarct size [73].

Hemodynamic and metabolic reserve

Patients with arterial occlusive disease are protected against ischemic episodes to a certain extent by compensatory mechanisms that help to prevent ischemia when perfusion pressure drops. This condition, studied by PET using ^{15}O-labeled tracers in patients with uni- or bilateral carotid artery disease [74], is indicated by regional vasodilatation manifesting itself as a focal increase in cerebral blood volume (CBV) in the supply territory of the occluded artery. Since a critical CBV distinguishing occluded from patent arterial territories could not be defined, the ratio of CBF to CBV was used as an indicator of local perfusion pressure. By calculating CBF/CBV (normal value = 10), territories of patent carotids, unilateral occlusion, occlusion with contralateral stenoses, and bilateral occlusions could be discriminated. Therefore, the quantity representing the reciprocal of the local mean vascular transit time is a measure of the perfusion reserve: the lower the value (from a normal value of 10 down to 5.5), the lower the flow velocity and the longer the residence time.

The lowest ratios were found in patients with symptoms suggestive of a hemodynamic rather than a thrombotic component to their ischemia, in whom maximal vasodilatation and low regional perfusion pressure may be expected. When the perfusion reserve is exhausted (i.e., at maximal vasodilatation), any further decrease in arterial input pressure produces a proportional decrease in both CBF and the CBF/CBV radio. In this condition of hemodynamic decompensation, the brain must draw upon the oxygen-carriage reserve to prevent energy failure and loss of function, as evidenced by an increase in the oxygen extraction ratio (OER) from the normal value of 40%–50% up to 85% [42,74]. Patients with low CBF/CBV and submaximal elevations of OER represent 10%–15% of the patients with cervical occlusive disease [74]; they exhibit the most advanced atherosclerotic lesions and their clinical symptoms are suggestive of hemodynamic ischemia. However, the relation between CBF/CBV ratios and OEF is rather variable, and CBF/CBV ratios alone only incompletely reflect hemodynamic impairment [75].

In a study of 30 medically treated patients with symptomatic carotid artery disease [76], the incidence of stroke was not related to perfusion reserve. Acetazolamide reactivity, determined by iodoamphetamine (IMP)-SPECT, was related to OEF and can be an indicator of hemodynamic failure [77]. Therefore, on the basis of such PET measurements, it is possible to discriminate patients with impaired hemodynamics, as well as to quantify the impairment of perfusion reserve using the CBF/CBV ratio. Additionally, patients can be identified who are in a more precarious physiologic state because their hemodynamic reserve is exhausted and their focal OER is increased. These two homeostatic mechanisms seem to act in series, thereby preventing a fall in $CMRO_2$ and, therefore, preventing functional disorder.

Estimation of prognosis

Correlation with outcome

The degree of functional recovery after an ischemic infarct of the brain is related to the location and size of the lesion; but neurons remaining within and in the neighborhood of the ischemic lesion, as well as compensatory mechanisms in functionally connected networks, may also contribute to the eventual outcome. Therefore, elucidating the effects of impaired interaction among brain regions and studying the mechanisms that reorganize destroyed networks as they relate to long-term prognosis is one of the most intriguing applications of functional imaging modalities. However, to date, only a few studies have looked at this issue. Kushner et al. observed a relation between size and severity of the initial metabolic disorder, judged by visual evaluation of PET scans and functional outcome in 36 stroke patients [69]. A normal PET or the presence of a mild metabolic abnormality was strongly associated with a good outcome or complete reversal of the neurologic dysfunction. Patients with moderate or severe metabolic abnormalities tended to have a stable disability or only moderate improvement. The only exceptions consisted of cases with a functionally relevant subcortical or lacunar infarct, in which relationships were not found in the concomitant CT results.

The significance of neuronal loss and functional deactivation to permanent neurologic deficits after ischemic stroke in peri-infarct tissue was demonstrated in 76 patients, in whom $rCMR_{glc}$ was measured in the subacute state (9 ± 7.2 days after the ictus) and related to the final outcome assessed by a rehabilitation index 50.5 ± 11.7 months after the stroke [78]. In the whole group, several variables – younger age, absence of arterial hypertension and cardiac disease, higher $rCMR_{glc}$ – were significantly related to better final outcome (p = 0.001). In addition, multiple regression analyses in homogeneous subgroups revealed a significant positive correlation of $rCMR_{glc}$ (p = 0.016) with recovery in hypertensive subjects, whereas age was the dominant prognostic factor in patients with normal blood pressure (p = 0.07). This result reflects the extent of hypertensive tissue damage outside the infarct and explains the subsequently reduced capacity to compensate for the focal ischemic insult.

Imaging recovery of motor function

The reorganization of the human motor system after stroke has been a focus of recent CBF PET studies [79,80], with most of these investigations performed in the chronic state after the attack. Ipsilateral activation of the motor cortex is consistently found to be stronger for movements of the paretic fingers after recovery from stroke, whereas movements of the unaffected hand (as in normal subjects) were accompanied mainly by activation of the contralateral cerebral cortex [81,82]. Chollet et al. reported that, in addition to stronger intensity, the spatial extent of activation in motor cortex was enlarged [81]. Somewhat increased activation on the ipsilateral side was also seen in the premotor and insular cortex. These results indicate that recruitment of ipsilateral cortices plays a role in recovery.

When activation patterns produced by movement of the affected hand in stroke victims were compared to those in normal volunteers [83], a significantly greater activation was found in patients in the ipsilateral premotor cortices and the contralateral cerebellum, as well as bilaterally in the lower parietal region and in the insula. Several authors described increased bilateral activation of the premotor cortex and supplementary motor area, often associated with anterior cingulate activation. This was the case with marked recovery of hand function after acute severe hemiparesis [84], and was also observed in patients with a permanent lesion in the internal capsule, who had suffered from acute hemiplegia and made a complete recovery from their motor deficit [85].

However, using an alternative motor task (thumb opposition), the different activation patterns observed – ipsilateral sensorimotor activation in only four of eight cases – made the role of the ipsilateral motor pathway controversial. Furthermore, a large ventral extension of the hand field of the contralateral sensorimotor cortex into the area normally associated with the face was detected in four cases with lesions in the posterior limb of the internal capsule. These results might be interpreted as a cortical adaptation to pyramidal tract disruption. Despite some controversial findings and the observations that ipsilateral activation was only seen in the most severely impaired patients [82] and that nonrecovered patients showed stronger ipsilateral and contralateral activation during passive movements than controls [86], these studies demonstrate that recovery of motor function is achieved by a redistribution of activity within a widespread network of parallel-acting motor areas and pathways.

This concept is supported by a multiple regression and discriminate analysis [87], which found a close relationship between $rCMR_{glc}$ of the bilateral SMA, ipsilateral thalamus, and contralateral cerebellum in recovered patients, suggesting a stronger functional association of these structures than in normal subjects or nonrecovered patients. In a related study, activation of a similar network, including bilateral occipital and bifrontal cortex, cerebellum, contralesional cingulate, hippocampus, and thalamus was statistically associated with recovery of motor function [88].

Prediction of prognosis in post-stroke aphasia

Studies of glucose metabolism after stroke have shown that the left temporoparietal cortex is crucial for language perception [71,89] and that the metabolic disturbance in these areas is related to outcome [90]. An investigation into the subacute state after stroke showed a highly significant correlation with language performance assessed at 2-year follow-up [91]. Receptive language disorder correlated with $rCMR_{glc}$ in the left temporal cortex and word fluency correlated with rCMR$_{glc}$ in the left prefrontal cortex. These results indicate that the functional disturbance, as measured by rCMR$_{glc}$ in speech-relevant brain regions soon after stroke, is predictive of the eventual outcome of aphasia.

It is not only functional deactivation (diaschisis) [63] that contributes to metabolic and perfusional changes in the neighborhood of the infarct: neuronal loss also plays a role. The condition of the surrounding tissue may affect the recovery of individual patients. On this basis, it is not surprising that, in patients with a poor outcome after post-stroke aphasia, metabolism in the hemisphere outside the infarct was significantly less than in those with good language recovery, indicating significant cell loss caused by the ischemic episode outside the ischemic core [90]. In addition, the functionality of the network was reduced in patients with an eventual poor outcome; during task performance, patients with an eventual good recovery predominantly activated structures in the ipsilateral hemisphere.

The involvement of various structures of the functional network in recovery from post-stroke aphasia can only be demonstrated by repeated activation studies at intervals after stroke. A few recent studies indicate that preserved left hemispheric speech areas are crucial for satisfactory outcome. Regional glucose metabolism at rest and during word repetition was studied by PET in six aphasic patients at 4 weeks and 12–18 months after the ischemic stroke [92]. Satisfactory recovery was related to activation of left hemispheric speech areas surrounding the infarct, especially the left superior temporal gyrus. Activation of right hemispheric regions was not efficacious for a considerable recovery from aphasia. Regional CBF PET studies showed left inferior temporal activation, but only a small right hemispheric response on a word retrieval task in six patients who had at least some recovery from aphasia [93].

Based on these preliminary data, language performance was related to ^{15}O-labeled water PET activation patterns in 23 right-handed aphasic patients 2 and 8 weeks after stroke [94]. In patients classified according to the site of lesion (frontal, n = 7; subcortical, n = 9; temporal, n = 7) and in 11 control subjects, flow changes caused by a word repetition task were calculated in 14 regions representing eloquent and contralateral homotopic areas, which were defined on coregistered MRI. Normal subjects showed a symmetric activation pattern of the superior temporal regions bilaterally and asymmetric activation in the inferior part of the left precentral gyrus and (with low intensity [4.13% relative difference]) in the left inferior frontal gyrus. In the three aphasic groups, the extent of recovery differed and was reflected in the activation pattern.

Patients with frontal and subcortical lesions improved substantially; they showed activation of the right inferior frontal gyrus and the right superior temporal gyrus during the first scan and had regained left superior temporal gyrus activation at follow-up. The temporal group improved only in word comprehension; they showed activation of the left area of Broca and supplementary motor areas in the first scan and had added the precentral gyrus bilaterally as well as the right superior temporal gyrus at follow-up, but the left superior temporal gyrus showed no activation. The shift of activation pattern necessary for satisfactory recovery could also be observed when frontal and subcortical groups were combined (because of their similar activation pattern and preservation of temporal structures) and subdivided into two subgroups, one with improvement of more than 50% and the other with improvement of less than 50% in Token test scores. Both subgroups exhibited a significant activation of the right inferior frontal gyrus in the first scan but not in the follow-up (see **Figure 5**). However, the group with >50% improvement had a significant activation of left temporal regions in the initial measurement, whereas the group with <50% improvement failed to activate these areas in either the first or second scans, despite the fact that these areas were morphologically intact.

Patients with destroyed left temporal language areas achieve the lowest grade of improvement and always incur a permanent deficit. The most striking compensatory mechanism in this group is activation of the left opercular region and the supplementary motor area for the task of word repetition during which these areas are either uninvolved or only slightly involved in normals. In the course of time, and with some improvement in comprehension, these patients activate right temporal and left frontal areas. In selected cases, these strategies can be partially successful in improving some language function [95], but, usually, the destruction of the left superior temporal gyrus prevents sufficient recovery of comprehension [96] and is associated with persistent impairment of repetition, naming, and sentence comprehension [97].

In summary, evidence extracted from these studies suggests a hierarchy within the language-related network regarding efficacy for improvement of aphasia, a conclusion also reached in recent reviews [98–100]. In the early period, some recovery might reflect the regression of diaschisis in areas that usually participate in language processing. In the long-term, outcome of aphasia is mainly dependent on the size and location of the left hemispheric lesion and the functional reorganization of the left hemisphere. If the more important left hemispheric areas are destroyed, the right hemispheric network can contribute to improvement to some extent [101]. However, satisfactory outcome and restoration of language function correlate with the possibility of activating left temporal areas.

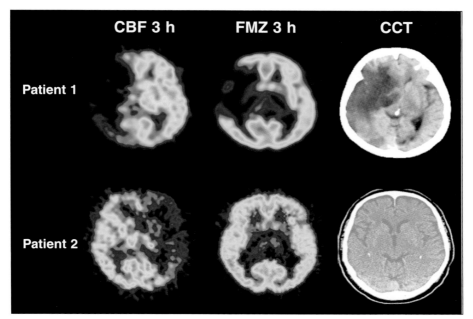

Figure 6. Effect of thrombolytic therapy on the use of perfusional disturbance and flumazenil (FMZ) binding as markers for neuronal integrity in two patients with large ischemic areas before initiation of treatment within the 3-hour window. In Patient 1, the large area with decreased FMZ binding predicts the corresponding large infarction on late cranial computed tomography (CCT). In Patient 2, FMZ binding within the normal range indicates intact morphology, as shown on late CCT infarction, and can be prevented by reperfusion induced by recombinant tissue plasminogen activator treatment. CBF: cerebral blood flow.

occasionally found in border zones of ischemia at the watershed between the anterior and middle cerebral arteries [129,130]. Such single cases may highlight the rationale for bypass surgery, by which flow and metabolism might be effectively increased [131–134]. However, Powers et al. [135] demonstrated that even patients with increased CBV/CBF on presurgical PET did not benefit clinically from EC-IC bypass: despite the fact that flow was improved and vasodilatation decreased in the revascularized regions, oxygen utilization was not affected. Overall, it must be concluded that this surgical procedure might be beneficial in only a few patients with a peculiar pathophysiologic pattern. The identification of these cases is extremely difficult, and therefore, a statistical proof of the therapeutic efficacy of this procedure cannot be easily achieved.

Conclusion

These few examples emphasize the important role of neuroimaging studies in providing surrogate markers for Phase II treatment trials in acute ischemic stroke.

Such studies can improve insight into the dependency of therapeutic effects on the pathophysiologic state of the tissue at a given time point after the onset of ischemia, and will help us to understand the striking differences in the efficacy of anti-ischemic therapy between animal models and human stroke.

References

1. Siesjö BK. Pathophysiology and treatment of focal cerebral ischemia. Part II: Mechanisms of damage and treatment. *J Neurosurg* 1992;77:337–54.
2. Pulsinelli W. Pathophysiology of acute ischaemic stroke. *Lancet* 1992;339:533–6.
3. Barone FC, Feuerstein GZ. Inflammatory mediators and stroke: new opportunities for novel therapeutics. *J Cereb Blood Flow Metab* 1999;19:819–34.
4. Schulz JB, Weller M, Moskowitz MA. Caspases as treatment targets in stroke and neurodegenerative diseases. *Ann Neurol* 1999;45:421–9.
5. Dirnagl U, Iadecola C, Moskowitz MA. Pathobiology of ischaemic stroke: an integrated view. *Trends Neurosci* 1999;22:391–7.
6. Heiss W-D. Experimental evidence of ischemic thresholds and functional recovery. *Stroke* 1992;23:1668–72.
7. Astrup J, Siesjo BK, Symon L. Thresholds in cerebral ischemia – the ischemic penumbra. *Stroke* 1981;12:723–5.
8. Phelps ME. Emission computed tomography. *Semin Nucl Med* 1977;7:337–65.
9. Ter-Pogossian MM. The origins of positron emission tomography. *Semin Nucl Med* 1992;22:140–9.
10. Wienhard K, Wagner R, Heiss WD. PET - Grundlagen und Anwendungen der PET. Berlin, Heidelberg, New York, London, Paris, Tokyo: Springer, 1989.
11. Wienhard K, Dahlbom M, Eriksson L et al. The ECAT EXACT HR: Performance of a new high resolution positron scanner. *J Comput Assist Tomogr* 1994;18:110–8.
12. Chatziioannou AF, Cherry SR, Shao Y et al. Performance evaluation of microPET: a high–resolution lutetium oxyorthosilicate PET scanner for animal imaging. *J Nucl Med* 1999;40(7):1164–75
13. Herscovitch P, Markham J, Raichle ME. Brain blood flow measured with intravenous $H_2^{15}O$. I. Theory and error analysis. *J Nucl Med* 1983;24:782–9.
14. Frackowiak RSJ, Lenzi G-L, Jones T et al. Quantitative measurement of regional cerebral blood flow and oxygen metabolism in man using ^{15}O and positron emission tomography: Theory, procedure, and normal values. *J Comput Assist Tomogr* 1980;4:727–36.
15. Sokoloff L. The relationship between function and energy metabolism: Its use in the localization of functional activity in the nervous system. *Neurosci Res Prog Bull* 1981;19:159–210.
16. Mintun MA, Raichle ME, Martin WRW et al. Brain oxygen utilization measured with O–15 radiotracers and positron emission tomography. *J Nucl Med* 1984;25:177–87.
17. Reivich M, Kuhl D, Wolf A et al. The [^{18}F]fluorodeoxyglucose method for the measurement of local cerebral glucose utilization in man. *Circ Res* 1979;44:127–37.
18. Phelps ME, Huang SC, Hoffman EJ et al. Tomographic measurement of local cerebral glucose metabolic rate in humans with (F-18)2-fluoro-2-deoxy-D-glucose: Validation of method. *Ann Neurol* 1979;6:371–88.
19. Sokoloff L, Reivich M, Kennedy C et al. The [^{14}C]-deoxyglucose method for the measurement of local cerebral glucose utilization: Theory, procedure, and normal values in the conscious and anesthetized albino rat. *J Neurochem* 1977;28:897–916.
20. Wienhard K, Pawlik G, Herholz K et al. Estimation of local cerebral glucose utilization by positron emission tomography of [^{18}F]2-fluoro-2-deoxy-D-glucose: a critical appraisal of optimization procedures. *J Cereb Blood Flow Metab* 1985;5:115–25.
21. Sette G, Baron JC, Young AR et al. In vivo mapping of brain benzodiazepine receptor changes by positron emission tomography after focal ischemia in the anesthetized baboon. *Stroke* 1993;24:2046–57.
22. Heiss W-D, Graf R, Fujita T et al. Early detection of irreversibly damaged ischemic tissue by flumazenil positron emission tomography in cats. *Stroke* 1997;28:2045–51.
23. Heiss W-D, Graf R. The ischemic penumbra. *Curr Opin Neurol* 1994;7:11–9.
24. Hossmann K-A. Viability thresholds and the penumbra of focal ischemia. *Ann Neurol* 1994;36:557–65.
25. Ginsberg MD, Pulsinelli WA. The ischemic penumbra, injury thresholds, and the therapeutic window for acute stroke. *Ann Neurol* 1994;36:553–4.

26. Baron JC, Rougemont D, Soussaline F et al. Local interrelationships of cerebral oxygen consumption and glucose utilization in normal subjects and in ischemic stroke patients: a positron tomography study. *J Cereb Blood Flow Metab* 1984;4:140–9.

27. De Reuck J, Stevens H, Jansen Heal. The significance of cobalt-55 positron emission tomography in ischemic stroke. *J Stroke Cerebrovasc Dis* 1999;8:17–21.

28. Mathias CJ, Welch MJ, Kilbourn MR et al. Radiolabeled hypoxic cell sensitizers: Tracers for assessment of ischemia. *Life Sci* 1987;41:199–206.

29. Yeh SH, Liu RS, Hu HH et al. Ischemic penumbra in acute stroke: demonstration by PET with fluorine-18 fluoromisonidazole. *J Nucl Med* 1994;35:205P.

30. Read SJ, Hirano T, Abbott DF et al. Identifying hypoxic tissue after acute ischemic stroke using PET and 18F-fluoromisonidazole. *Neurology* 1998;51:1617–21.

31. Tenjin H, Ueda S, Mizukawa N et al. Positron emission tomographic measurement of acute hemodynamic changes in primate middle cerebral artery occlusion. *Neurol Med Chir (Tokyo)* 1992;32:805–10.

32. Pappata S, Fiorelli M, Rommel T et al. PET study of changes in local brain hemodynamics and oxygen metabolism after unilateral middle cerebral artery occlusion in baboons. *J Cereb Blood Flow Metab* 1993;13:416–24.

33. Heiss W-D, Graf R, Wienhard K et al. Dynamic penumbra demonstrated by sequential multitracer PET after middle cerebral artery occlusion in cats. *J Cereb Blood Flow Metab* 1994;14:892–902.

34. Heiss W-D, Graf R, Löttgen J et al. Repeat positron emission tomographic studies in transient middle cerebral artery occlusion in cats: residual perfusion and efficacy of postischemic reperfusion. *J Cereb Blood Flow Metab* 1997;17:388–400.

35. Heiss W-D, Rosner G. Functional recovery of cortical neurons as related to degree and duration of ischemia. *Ann Neurol* 1983;14:294–301.

36. Kuhl DE, Phelps ME, Kowell AP et al. Effects of stroke on local cerebral metabolism and perfusion: Mapping by emission computed tomography of ^{18}FDG and ^{13}NH$_3$. *Ann Neurol* 1980;8:47–60.

37. Baron JC, Frackowiak RS, Herholz K et al. Use of PET methods for measurement of cerebral energy metabolism and hemodynamics in cerebrovascular disease. *J Cereb Blood Flow Metab* 1989;9:723–42.

38. Powers WJ, Grubb RL Jr, Darriet D et al. Cerebral blood flow and cerebral metabolic rate of oxygen requirements for cerebral function and viability in humans. *J Cereb Blood Flow Metab* 1985;5:600–8.

39. Baron JC, Bousser MG, Rey A et al. Reversal of focal "misery-perfusion syndrome" by extra-intracranial arterial bypass in hemodynamic cerebral ischemia. A case study with ^{15}O positron emission tomography. *Stroke* 1981;12:454–9.

40. Ackerman RH, Correia JA, Alpert NM et al. Positron imaging in ischemic stroke disease using compounds labeled with oxygen 15. Initial results of clinicophysiologic correlations. *Arch Neurol* 1981;38:537–43.

41. Hakim AM, Evans AC, Berger L et al. The effect of nimodipine on the evolution of human cerebral infarction studied by PET. *J Cereb Blood Flow Metab* 1989;9:523–34.

42. Powers WJ, Press GA, Grubb RL Jr et al. The effect of hemodynamically significant carotid artery disease on the hemodynamic status of the cerebral circulation. *Ann Intern Med* 1987;106:27–35.

43. Baron JC. Mapping the ischaemic penumbra with PET: implications for acute stroke treatment. *Cerebrovasc Dis* 1999;9:193–201.

44. Marchal G, Beaudouin V, Rioux P et al. Prolonged persistence of substantial volumes of potentially viable brain tissue after stroke. A correlative PET-CT study with voxel based data analysis. *Stroke* 1996;27:599–606.

45. Heiss W-D, Huber M, Fink GR et al. Progressive derangement of periinfarct viable tissue in ischemic stroke. *J Cereb Blood Flow Metab* 1992;12:193–203.

46. Yamauchi H, Fukuyama H, Nagahama Y et al. Evidence of misery perfusion and risk for recurrent stroke in major cerebral arterial occlusive diseases from PET. *J Neurol Neurosurg Psychiatry* 1996;61:18–25.

47. Wise RJS, Bernardi S, Frackowiak RSJ et al. Serial observations on the pathophysiology of acute stroke. The transition from ischaemia to infarction as reflected in regional oxygen extraction. *Brain* 1983;106:197–222.

48. Heiss W-D, Fink GR, Huber M et al. Positron emission tomography imaging and the therapeutic window. *Stroke* 1993;24:I50–I53.

49. Furlan M, Marchal G, Viader F et al. Spontaneous neurological recovery after stroke and the fate of the ischemic penumbra. *Ann Neurol* 1996;40:216–26.

50. Heiss W-D, Grond M, Thiel A et al. Permanent cortical damage detected by flumazenil positron emission tomography in acute stroke. *Stroke* 1998;29:454–61.

51. Heiss W-D, Thiel A, Grond M et al. Which targets are relevant for therapy of acute ischemic stroke? *Stroke* 1999;30:1486–9.

52. Heiss W-D, Kracht LW, Thiel A et al. Penumbral probability thresholds of cortical flumazenil binding and blood flow predicting tissue outcome in patients with cerebral ischaemia. *Brain* 2001;124:20–9.

53. Wise RJS, Rhodes CG, Gibbs JM et al. Disturbance of oxidative metabolism of glucose in recent human cerebral infarcts. *Ann Neurol* 1983;14:627–37.

54. Berkelbach van der Sprenkel JW, Luyten PR, van Rijen PC et al. Cerebral lactate detected by regional proton magnetic resonance spectroscopy in a patient with cerebral infarction. *Stroke* 1988;19:1556–60.

55. Bruhn H, Frahm J, Gyngell ML et al. Cerebral metabolism in man after acute stroke: new observations using localized proton NMR spectroscopy. *Magn Reson Med* 1989;9:126–31.

56. Lanfermann H, Kugel H, Heindel W et al. Metabolic changes in acute and subacute cerebral infarctions: findings at proton MR spectroscopic imaging. *Radiology* 1995;196:203–10.

57. Ramsay SC, Weiller C, Myers R et al. Monitoring by PET of macrophage accumulation in brain after ischemic stroke. *Lancet* 1992;339:1054–5.

58. Wang PY, Kao CH, Mui MY et al. Leukocyte infiltration in acute hemispheric ischemic stroke. *Stroke* 1993;24:236–40.

59. Baron JC, Bouser MG, Comar D et al. "Crossed cerebellar diaschisis" in human supratentorial brain infarction. *Ann Neurol* 1980;8:128.

60. Miura H, Nagata K, Hirata Y et al. Evolution of crossed cerebellar diaschisis in middle cerebral artery infarction. *J Neuroimaging* 1994;4:91–6.

61. Pawlik G, Herholz B, Beil C et al. Remote effects of focal lesions on cerebral blood flow and metabolism. In: Heiss W-D, editor. *Functional Mapping of the Brain in Vascular Disorders*. Berlin, Heidelberg, New York, Tokyo: Springer, 1985:59–84.

62. Mies G, Auer LM, Ebhardt G et al. Flow and neuronal density in tissue surrounding chronic infarction. *Stroke* 1983;14:22–7.

63. Feeney DM, Baron JC. Diaschisis. *Stroke* 1986;17:817–30.

64. Kushner M, Alavi A, Reivich M et al. Contralateral cerebellar hypometabolism following cerebral insult: a positron emission tomographic study. *Ann Neurol* 1984;15:425–34.

65. Martin WRW, Raichle ME. Cerebellar blood flow and metabolism in cerebral hemisphere infarction. *Ann Neurol* 1983;14:168–76.

66. Szelies B, Herholz K, Pawlik G et al. Widespread functional effects of discrete thalamic infarction. *Arch Neurol* 1991;48:178–82.

67. Baron JC, Levasseur M, Mazoyer B et al. Thalamocortical diaschisis: positron emission tomography in humans. *J Neurol Neurosurg Psychiatry* 1992;55:935–42.

68. Reivich M. Crossed cerebellar diaschisis. *Am J Neuroradiol* 1992;13:62–4.

69. Kushner M, Reivich M, Fieschi C et al. Metabolic and clinical correlates of acute ischemic infarction. *Neurology* 1987;37:1103–10.

70. Metter EJ, Kempler D, Jackson C et al. Cerebral glucose metabolism in Wernicke's, Broca's, and conduction aphasia. *Arch Neurol* 1989;46:27–34.

71. Karbe H, Herholz K, Szelies B et al. Regional metabolic correlates of Token test results in cortical and subcortical left hemispheric infarction. *Neurology* 1989;39:1083–8.

72. Tanaka M, Kondo S, Hirai S et al. Crossed cerebellar diaschisis accompanied by hemiataxia: a PET study. *J Neurol Neurosurg Psychiatry* 1992;55:121–5.

73. Serrati C, Marchal G, Rioux P et al. Contralateral cerebellar hypometabolism: a predictor for stroke outcome. *J Neurol Neurosurg Psychiatry* 1994;57:174–9.

74. Gibbs JM, Wise RJ, Leenders KL et al. Evaluation of cerebral perfusion reserve in patients with carotid-artery occlusion. *Lancet* 1984;1:310–4.

75. Itoh M, Hatazawa J, Pozzilli C et al. Haemodynamics and oxygen metabolism in patients after reversible ischaemic attack of minor ischaemic stroke assessed with positron emission tomography. *Neuroradiology* 1987;29:416–21.

76. Powers WJ, Tempel LW, Grubb RL, Jr. Influence of cerebral hemodynamics on stroke risk: one-year follow-up of 30 medically treated patients. *Ann Neurol* 1989;25:325–30.

77. Hirano T, Minematsu K, Hasegawa Y et al. Acetazolamide reactivity on ^{123}I-IMP single photon emission computed tomography in patients with major cerebral artery occlusive disease: correlation with positron emission tomography parameters. *J Cereb Blood Flow Metab* 1994;14:763–70.

78. Heiss W-D, Emunds HG, Herholz K. Cerebral glucose metabolism as a predictor of rehabilitation after ischemic stroke. *Stroke* 1993;24:1784–8.

79. Chollet F, Weiller C. Imaging recovery of function following brain injury. *Curr Opin Neurobiol* 1994;4:226–30.

80. Weiller C. Recovery from motor stroke: human positron emission tomography studies. *Cerebrovasc Dis* 1995;5:282–91.

81. Chollet F, Di Piero V, Wise RJS et al. The functional anatomy of motor recovery after stroke in humans: a study with positron emission tomography. *Ann Neurol* 1991;29:63–71.

82. Weder B, Seitz RJ. Deficient cerebral activation pattern in stroke recovery. *Neuroreport* 1994;5:457–60.

83. Weiller C, Chollet F, Friston KJ et al. Functional reorganization of the brain in recovery from striatocapsular infarction in man. *Ann Neurol* 1992;31:463–72.

84. Seitz RJ, Hoflich P, Binkofski F et al. Role of the premotor cortex in recovery from middle cerebral artery infarction. *Arch Neurol* 1998;55:1081–8.

85. Weiller C, Ramsay SC, Wise RJS et al. Individual patterns of functional reorganization in the human cerebral cortex after capsular infarction. *Ann Neurol* 1993;33:181–9.

86. Nelles G, Spiekermann G, Jueptner M et al. Reorganization of sensory and motor systems in hemiplegic stroke patients. A positron emission tomography study. *Stroke* 1999;30:1510–6.

87. Azari NP, Binkofski F, Pettigrew KD et al. Enhanced regional cerebral metabolic interactions in thalamic circuitry predicts motor recovery in hemiparetic stroke. *Hum Brain Mapp* 1996;4:240–53.

88. Seitz RJ, Azari NP, Knorr U et al. The role of diaschisis in stroke recovery. *Stroke* 1999;30:1844–50.

89. Metter EJ. Neuroanatomy and physiology of aphasia: evidence from positron emission tomography. *Aphasiology* 1987;1:3–33.

90. Heiss W-D, Kessler J, Karbe H et al. Cerebral glucose metabolism as a predictor of recovery from aphasia in ischemic stroke. *Arch Neurol* 1993;50:958–64.

91. Karbe H, Kessler J, Herholz K et al. Long-term prognosis of poststroke aphasia studied with positron emission tomography. *Arch Neurol* 1995;52:186–90.

92. Heiss W-D, Karbe H, Weber-Luxenburger G et al. Speech-induced cerebral metabolic activation reflects recovery from aphasia. *J Neurol Sci* 1997;145:213–7.

93. Warburton E, Price CJ, Swinburn K et al. Mechanisms of recovery from aphasia: evidence from positron emission tomography studies. *J Neurol Neurosurg Psychiatry* 1999;66:155–61.

94. Heiss W-D, Kessler J, Thiel A et al. Differential capacity of left and right hemispheric areas for compensation of poststroke aphasia. *Ann Neurol* 1999;45:430–8.

95. Weiller C, Isensee C, Rijntjes M et al. Recovery from Wernicke's aphasia: a positron emission tomographic study. *Ann Neurol* 1995;37:723–32.

96. Naeser MA, Gaddie A, Palumbo CL et al. Late recovery of auditory comprehension in global aphasia. Improved recovery observed with subcortical temporal isthmus lesion vs Wernicke's cortical area lesion. *Arch Neurol* 1990;47:425–32.

97. Selnes OA, Knopman DS, Niccum N et al. The critical role of Wernicke's area in sentence repetition. *Ann Neurol* 1985;17:549–57.

98. Ferro JM, Mariano G, Madureira S. Recovery from aphasia and neglect. *Cerebrovasc Dis* 1999;9(Suppl. 5):6–22.

99. Samson Y, Belin P, Zilbovicius M et al. Mécanismes de la récupération de l'aphasie et imagerie cérébrale. *Rev Neurol (Paris)* 1999;155:725–30.

100. Khatri P, Hier DB. Imaging aphasia: the coming paradigm shift. *Brain Cogn* 2000;42:60–3.

101. Gainotti G. The riddle of the right hemisphere's contribution to the recovery of language. *Eur J Disord Commun* 1993;28:227–46.

102. Kertesz A, Lau WK, Polk M. The structural determinants of recovery in Wernicke's aphasia. *Brain Lang* 1993;44:153–64.

103. Kessler J, Thiel A, Karbe H et al. Piracetam improves activated blood flow and facilitates rehabilitation of poststroke aphasic patients. *Stroke* 2000;31:2112–6.

104. De Keyser J, Sulter G, Luiten PG. Clinical trials with neuroprotective drugs in acute ischaemic stroke: are we doing the right thing? *Trends Neurosci* 1999;22:535–40.

105. Baron JC, von Kummer R, del Zoppo GJ. Treatment of acute ischemic stroke. Challenging the concept of a rigid and universal time window. *Stroke* 1995;26:2219–21.

106. Hakim AM. Hemodynamic and metabolic studies in stroke. *Semin Neurol* 1989;9:286–92.

107. Fisher M. Characterizing the target of acute stroke therapy. *Stroke* 1997;28:866–72.

108. Saver JL, Johnston KC, Homer D et al. Infarct volume as a surrogate or auxiliary outcome measure in ischemic stroke clinical trials. The RANTTAS Investigators. *Stroke* 1999;30:293–8.

109. The NINDS rt–PA Stroke Study Group. Tissue plasminogen activator for acute ischemic stroke. *N Engl J Med* 1995;333:1581–7.

110. Hacke W, Kaste M, Fieschi C et al. Intravenous thrombolysis with recombinant tissue plasminogen activator for acute hemispheric stroke. The European Cooperative Acute Stroke Study (ECASS). *JAMA* 1995;274:1017–25.

111. Hacke W, Kaste M, Fieschi C et al. Randomised double-blind placebo-controlled trial of thrombolytic therapy with intravenous alteplase in acute ischemic stroke (ECASS II). *Lancet* 1998;352:1245–51.

112. Furlan A, Higashida R, Wechsler L et al. Intra-arterial prourokinase for acute ischemic stroke. The PROACT II study: A randomized controlled trial. *JAMA* 1999;282:2003–11.

113. Heiss W-D. Ischemic penumbra: evidence from functional imaging in man. *J Cereb Blood Flow Metab* 2000;20:1276–93.

114. Heiss W-D, Grond M, Thiel A et al. Tissue at risk of infarction rescued by early reperfusion: a positron emission tomography study in systemic recombinant tissue plasminogen activator thrombolysis of acute stroke. *J Cereb Blood Flow Metab* 1998;18:1298–1307.

115. Marks MP, Decrespigny A, Lentz D et al. Acute and chronic stroke: navigated spin-echo diffusion-weighted MR imaging. *Radiology* 1996;199:403–8.

116. Kidwell CS, Alger JR, Di Salle F et al. Diffusion MRI in patients with transient ischemic attacks. *Stroke* 1999;30:1174–80.

117. Kidwell CS, Saver JL, Mattiello J et al. Thrombolytic reversal of acute human cerebral ischemic injury shown by diffusion/perfusion magnetic resonance imaging. *Ann Neurol* 2000;47:462–9.

118. Heiss W-D, Kracht L, Grond M et al. Early [^{11}C]Flumazenil/H$_2$O positron emission tomography predicts irreversible ischemic cortical damage in stroke patients receiving acute thrombolytic therapy. *Stroke* 2000;31:366–9.

119. Mohr JP, Orgogozo JM, Harrison MJG et al. Meta-analysis of oral nimodipine trials in acute ischemic stroke. *Cerebrovasc Dis* 1994;4:197–203.

120. Heiss W-D, Holthoff V, Hartmann-Klosterkötter U et al. Nimodipine improves glucose metabolism after stroke. *Stroke* 1990;21:I158–I159.

121. Huber M, Kittner B, Hojer C et al. Effect of propentofylline on regional cerebral glucose metabolism in acute ischemic stroke. *J Cereb Blood Flow Metab* 1993;13:526–30.

122. Yamauchi H, Fukuyama H, Ogawa M et al. Hemodilution improves cerebral hemodynamics in internal carotid artery occlusion. *Stroke* 1993;24:1885–90.

123. Hsu CY, Faught RE Jr, Furlan AJ et al. Intravenous prostacyclin in acute nonhemorrhagic stroke: A placebo-controlled double-blind trial. *Stroke* 1987;18:352–8.

124. Heiss W-D, Pawlik G, Hebold I et al. Can PET estimate functional recovery and indicate therapeutic strategy in stroke? In: Krieglstein J, editor. *Pharmacology of Cerebral Ischemia*. Stuttgart: Wiss. Verlagsges, 1989:433–8.

125. Argentino C, Toni D, Sacchetti ML et al. Hemodilution and monosialoganglioside GM1 in the treatment of acute ischemic stroke. In: Krieglstein J, editor. *Pharmacology of Cerebral Ischemia 1988*. Stuttgart: Wiss. Verlagsges, 1989:449–53.

126. The EC/IC Bypass Study Group. Failure of extracranial-intracranial arterial bypass to reduce the risk of ischemic stroke. Results of an international randomized trial. *N Engl J Med* 1985;313:1191–200.

127. Gibbs JM, Wise RJS, Thomas DJ et al. Cerebral haemodynamic changes after extracranial-intracranial bypass surgery. *J Neurol Neurosurg Psychiatry* 1987;50:140–50.

128. Yamauchi H, Fukuyama H, Fujimoto N et al. Significance of low perfusion with increased oxygen extraction fraction in a case of internal carotid artery stenosis. *Stroke* 1992;23:431–2.

129. Leblanc R, Yamamoto YL, Tyler JL et al. Borderzone ischemia. *Ann Neurol* 1987;22:707–13.

130. Carpenter DA, Grubb RL Jr, Powers WJ. Borderzone hemodynamics in cerebrovascular disease. *Neurology* 1990;40:1587–92.

131. Nagata S, Fujii K, Matsushima T et al. Evaluation of EC-IC bypass for patients with atherosclerotic occlusive cerebrovascular disease: clinical and positron emission tomographic studies. *Neurol Res* 1991;13:209–16.

132. Ishikawa T, Yasui N, Suzuki A et al. STA-MCA bypass surgery for internal carotid artery occlusion - comparative follow-up study. *Neurol Med Chir* 1992;32:5–9.

133. Ogawa A, Kameyama M, Muraishi K et al. Cerebral blood flow and metabolism following superficial temporal artery to superior cerebellar artery bypass for vertebrobasilar occlusive disease. *J Neurosurg* 1992;76:955–60.

134. Muraishi K, Kameyama M, Sato K et al. Cerebral circulatory and metabolic changes following EC/IC bypass surgery in cerebral occlusive diseases. *Neurol Res* 1993;15:97–103.

135. Powers WJ, Martin WRH, Herscovitch P et al. Extracranial-intracranial bypass surgery: Hemodynamic and metabolic effects. *Neurology* 1984;34:1168–74.

8

Recovery and plasticity imaging in stroke patients

Joachim Liepert & Cornelius Weiller

Introduction

Within the last two decades, the conceptual view of the organization of the human brain has changed remarkably. In the early 1980s, the ability of the adult brain to adapt to lesions in the peripheral or central nervous system was demonstrated in animals [1–10]. Use-dependent modulations of brain organization have also been reported [11–13]. Plastic changes have been described in the cortex [5,11,12,14,15], thalamus and brainstem [16–18], and can be associated with chemical factors, e.g., neurotransmitters such as glutamate [19–22], gamma amino butyric acid (GABA) [23–29], norepinephrine [30], and acetylcholine [31]. In addition, neurotrophins, e.g., brain-derived neurotrophic factor (BDNF), are upregulated following brain injury [32–34] and dendritic branching may occur [35–38].

After a stroke, most patients develop at least some recovery of function. In the majority of cases these improvements occur within the first 3 months after the injury. The mechanisms leading to good recovery in some and poor recovery in others are only partially understood. Lesion size, for example, is of minor importance [39]. In contrast, lesion location and the amount of corticospinal tract destruction are more critical. It is important to learn more about brain areas involved in recovery processes to predict *a priori* which patient may benefit from rehabilitation, and to develop specific rehabilitative strategies for individual subjects.

Today, various imaging techniques are available that allow identification of neuronal network reorganization in the human brain *in vivo*. Knowledge regarding the capacity of the brain for neuronal reorganization not only improves our understanding of how the brain works but, even more importantly, could also have major implications for the development of adequate therapeutic strategies.

Brain plasticity can be defined as the ability of the brain to reorganize itself [40]. Following a lesion, there are at least four different mechanisms by which plastic changes may be evoked:

1. passive adaptation of the brain to the lesion and the impairment of neuronal networks, e.g., diaschisis [41]

2. reorganization of the brain due to spontaneous recovery of (partially) damaged brain tissue

3. reorganization induced by behavioral consequences of the lesion, e.g., learned nonuse of a formerly paretic limb

4. reorganization of the brain evoked by specific therapeutic interventions

Depending on the time course after stroke, there may be a considerable overlap between these different mechanisms. However, identification of the predominant condition is desirable for an appropriate therapeutic approach. For example, patients with a learned nonuse of the affected limb should be treated with a combination of behavioral and intense physical therapy.

Imaging techniques

The most important techniques used to visualize brain plasticity are functional magnetic resonance imaging (fMRI), positron emission tomography (PET) with a $[^{15}O]$ H_2O tracer, magnetoencephalography (MEG), electroencephalography (EEG), transcranial Doppler ultrasound (TCD), and transcranial magnetic stimulation (TMS).

fMRI and PET can demonstrate changes of regional blood flow in the brain. These blood flow modulations are thought to correspond to changes of neuronal activity. The main advantage of fMRI and PET is that the exact localization of regional blood flow changes in the whole brain can be ascertained. Major disadvantages of these techniques are the limitations in the resolution of time sequences, high expense of each examination, and limited availability of PET scanners and radioactive tracers.

EEG and MEG recordings reflect 'true' neuronal activity (in contrast to blood flow changes) and have an excellent resolution in the time domain, but spatial resolution is limited, particularly for localization of deep, subcortical sources. MEG machines are expensive and only accessible at specialized centers. EEG recordings allow identification of radially and tangentially oriented dipoles. In contrast, identification of radially oriented dipoles by MEG is very limited.

TCD and TMS are the least expensive imaging techniques discussed and are ideally suited for follow-up investigations. Blood flow changes detected by TCD can be employed to indicate modifications of neuronal activity. However, TCD does not allow a precise localization of the brain areas undergoing plastic changes since TCD mainly monitors blood flow in large, but not in small, cerebral vessels. TMS allows one to investigate the integrity of the corticospinal motor tracts and to study various aspects of motor excitability, e.g., excitatory and inhibitory circuits in the human motor cortex [42]. TMS mapping techniques enable one to explore the cortical representation area size of various muscles. A main advantage is that TMS investigations are independent of the subject's motor performance ability. In addition, with repetitive TMS it is possible to detect functionally relevant brain areas by temporarily modifying their activity; this is not limited to the motor domain [43].

The most appropriate way to reveal brain adaptations after a lesion, or during recovery of function, is a combination of different techniques, e.g., fMRI with TMS and EEG/MEG recordings. Such a complementary arrangement would have high spatial and temporal resolution, allow the evaluation of neuronal excitability, and may help in assessing the functional significance of brain reorganization.

Reorganization and restoration of function

The exact relationship between reorganization and restoration of function is not known. In stroke patients, PET data can show enhanced activation in the uninjured hemisphere with [44] or without concomitant improvement in motor function (see **Figure 1**) [45]. Patients with peripheral facial nerve palsy (Bell's palsy) may exhibit enlarged hand muscle-evoked representations without obvious improvement of hand motor performance [46], and patients with hemifacial spasm may show a decreased hand representation without restriction of hand function in everyday life [47]. The latter two examples of reorganization can be interpreted as examples of the competitiveness inherent to the brain.

Reorganization may be harmful. In amputees, a positive correlation has been described between the amount of cortical reorganization and the intensity of phantom pain [48,49]. Restitution of lost or impaired function can be related to a recovery of partially damaged tissue, or can be the result of recruitment of new neuronal circuits. Plastic changes may include a modified balance between

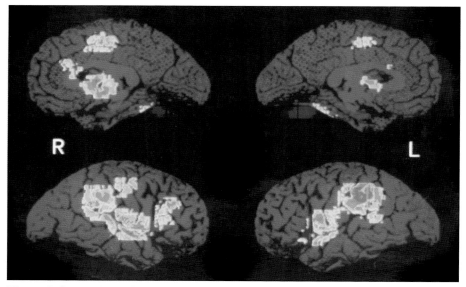

Figure 1. Comparison of differences in activation between 10 patients with striatocapsular infarcts and 10 normal subjects. Positron emission tomography (PET) was performed during movements of the affected hand (right hand). Patients exhibit stronger activations in the non-lesioned hemisphere ipsilateral to the affected hand and a lateral extension of the hand area in the damaged hemisphere (With kind permission from Weiller et al. [44]).

inhibitory and excitatory networks to achieve disinhibition. In addition, undamaged circuits could also contribute to achieve impaired behavioral goals [50].

The degree to which brain areas can be recruited for reorganization after an infarction is probably influenced by numerous factors, e.g., site and extent of the lesion, remote lesion-induced effects in structurally intact areas ('diaschisis'), and prestroke organization of motor areas (e.g., number of ipsilateral, uncrossed corticospinal fibers) [51].

Motor and somatosensory reorganization

fMRI/PET findings

Studies on sensorimotor reorganization after stroke show a number of congruencies, but also several substantial differences (see **Table 1**). In most fMRI or PET studies involving active or passive movements, a widespread network of neurons was activated in both hemispheres. The areas included frontal and parietal cortices, and sometimes the basal ganglia and cerebellum, in accordance with the finding that various brain areas are devoted to motor control and motor activity [83]. In particular, (ipsilateral) premotor cortex, supplementary motor area (SMA), anterior parts of the insula/frontal operculum, and bilateral inferior parietal cortices are often activated [44,45,52,58,61,65,69,77,82,84,88,92]. These results suggest that sensorimotor functions are represented in extended, variable, probably parallel processing, bilateral networks [98,99]. Historically, some of these areas (e.g., SMA, lateral premotor cortex) were believed to be involved in planning, preparation, and initiation of movements. However, these additional motor areas contribute substantial numbers of fibers to the corticospinal tract [100,101] and could functionally substitute for damaged fibers.

During finger movement, stroke patients usually show stronger activations compared to healthy controls. This could reflect a greater effort to perform the movement [102]. Alternative explanations might be a lesion-induced disinhibition [103–106] through impairment of transcallosal fibers, or a compensatory brain mechanism attempting to enhance excitability through reduction of intracortical inhibition.

Contributions from the nonlesioned hemisphere

Another common finding is the activation of areas in the undamaged hemisphere. Again, the interpretation of this result is crucial. In some, but not all studies, these activations could be related to the occurrence of associated movements of the unaffected hand. In several experiments, TMS was used to correlate the occurrence of motor-evoked potentials (MEPs) with clinical outcome after stimulation of the ipsilateral, nonlesioned hemisphere. Caramia et al. described patients who had an early and rapid recovery [107]. In these patients, MEPs could be produced by ipsilateral TMS in the recovered hand. However, several studies have reported a correlation between ipsilaterally produced MEPs and a poor outcome [108,109]. Palmer et al. did not find any evidence for the involvement of ipsilateral fast corticospinal pathways in recovery from stroke [110].

In summary, it seems possible that two different patient groups exist: one small group (the minority) with a larger portion of ipsilateral, uncrossed corticospinal fibers that contribute to a quick recovery; and the majority, probably with fewer ipsilateral corticospinal connections. These may become accessible (possibly due to an intracortical disinhibition) but may not substantially support restitution of function. Therefore, ipsilateral activations observed in fMRI or PET are not necessarily a main cause for clinical restitution. Feydy et al. [95] described a potentially important finding: they observed two different patterns of activation after stroke and suggested that persisting activity in the nonlesioned hemisphere was associated with primary motor cortex lesions in the other hemisphere. The other pattern consisted of enhanced activations in the affected hemisphere and occurred in patients with lesions outside the primary motor cortex.

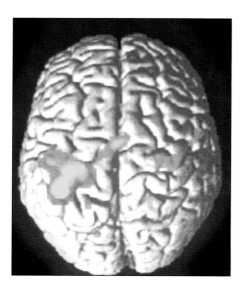

Figure 2. Functional magnetic resonance imaging results in a patient who had suffered a stroke 1 year ago and participated in a 12-day trial of constraint-induced movement therapy (CIMT). Activations obtained during movements of the paretic hand are shown: red signifies areas activated exclusively prior to CIMT; yellow signifies areas activated before and after CIMT; and green signifies areas activated exclusively after CIMT. Following CIMT, the activation pattern in the lesioned hemisphere shifted anteriorly, the supplementary motor area activation was enlarged, and additional activations were found in the nonlesioned hemisphere. (Dr F Hamzei, personal communication, with permission).

Another limitation in many studies is that stroke patients are enrolled after substantial recovery of function. This makes an interpretation even more difficult, as it remains unclear whether the activations represent a correlate of recovery or if they are related to epiphenomena. To evaluate the contribution of the undamaged hemisphere, studies are needed that correlate activations in specific brain areas with a change in motor performance. This can be done by repetition of measurements during spontaneous recovery [59,64,76,77,83–85, 92,95,97] or after a particular therapeutic intervention (see **Figure 2**) [66,75,80,81,86–88,94].

TMS findings

A large proportion of these studies was performed with TMS and indicated a reorganization of hand muscle representations in the affected hemisphere (see **Figures 3**, **4**, and **5**) [59,64,66,67,80,81,87,110]. Similar results were also reported in PET and fMRI studies [77,82,88,89,94]. In contrast, recovery of tongue muscle paresis and dysphagia seems to be mediated by the nonlesioned hemisphere [76,111].

Another approach to evaluate the functional significance of activations observed in PET or fMRI is the use of repetitive TMS (rTMS) [112]. In a group of blind Braille readers, Cohen et al. demonstrated that rTMS over the occipital cortex impaired the ability to read Braille [43]. Walsh et al. [113] showed that TMS over right parietal cortex areas impaired visual conjunction search. TMS over human visual area V_5 modified visual perception [114]. Therefore, rTMS applied over activated areas should have some impact on performance if these activations are

Author	Technique	Patients and recovery: good/partially/poor	Task	Results
Chollet et al., 1991 [52]	PET (H₂¹⁵O)	6/0/0	Active finger movements	Recovered hand: rCBF increases in both sensorimotor cortices, both cerebellar hemispheres, insula, parietal and premotor cortices
Weiller et al., 1992 [44]	PET (H₂¹⁵O)	Striatocapsular lesions 10/0/0	Active finger movements	Recovered hand: greater activation than normal in both insulae, inferior parietal, prefrontal and anterior cingulate, ipsilateral premotor cortex and basal ganglia, and contralateral cerebellum
Weiller et al., 1993 [53]	PET (H₂¹⁵O)	Striatocapsular lesions 8/0/0	Active finger movements	Recovered hand: contralateral sensorimotor cortex, SMA, insula, frontal operculum, parietal cortex
Weder et al., 1994 [54]	PET	Subcortical lesions 5 patients	Tactile exploration	Main activations in contralateral sensorimotor cortex, poor performance: low rCBF in contralateral SM1 at rest, and bilateral activation of SM1 during task performance
Weder & Seitz, 1994 [55]	PET	Good motor function, impaired tactile discrimination	Tactile discrimination	Deficient activations in SMA, parietal, premotor and midfrontal areas
Binkofski et al., 1996 [56]	PET (glucose)	23 stroke patients		Poor motor recovery was associated with reduced thalamic metabolism and more severe damage to the pyramidal tract
Iglesias et al., 1996 [57]	PET (H₂¹⁵O)	30 patients, measured 18 h and 15–30 days after stroke		Oxygen consumption in the nonlesioned hemisphere was not correlated with the initial clinical deficit. No evidence for a role of the nonlesioned hemisphere in early recovery
Pantano et al., 1996 [58]	SPECT	37, chronic stroke	Active finger movements	Severe motor deficit: low rCBF in SMA and parietal area of damaged hemisphere. Motor improvement: rCBF increases in basal ganglia and premotor cortex of undamaged hemisphere
Cicinelli et al., 1997 [59]	TMS mapping	10 patients with subcortical and 8 patients with cortical lesions, examined approximately 8 weeks and 16 weeks after infarct		Initially smaller motor output area in the lesioned hemisphere, significant enlargement after 8 weeks. Anomalously located most excitable scalp sites in patients (both hemispheres)
Cramer et al., 1997 [60]	fMRI	5 patients with subcortical and 5 patients with cortical lesions 10/0/0	Finger tapping	Activation of same motor areas as controls, but to a larger extent, particularly in the nonlesioned hemisphere
Dettmers et al., 1997 [61]	PET (H₂O)	6 patients with moderate to good recovery	Key presses with different degrees of force	Force exertion induced less activation in patients than in normals. Correlation between rCBF and increasing forces was logarithmic in normals and polynomial in patients. In patients, ipsilateral parts of SMA, dorsolateral premotor, insular and parietal areas were additionally activated

Table 1. Imaging studies of motor and somatosensory areas after stroke.

Author	Technique	Patients and recovery: good/partially/poor	Task	Results
Honda et al., 1997 [62]	PET + MRP	2 patients with cortical + subcortical lesion 2/0/0	Active hand movements	Recovered hand: movement-related cortical potential without contralateral predominance. PET: increased rCBF in ipsilateral, undamaged hemisphere. Undamaged hemisphere especially important prior to movement onset
Juhasz et al., 1997 [63]	EEG	40 patients, studied in acute phase and after recovery		In subcortical lesions, alpha peak frequency was decreased in the affected hemisphere (acute stage), and normalized after recovery. In territorial strokes, alpha peak frequency was reduced bilaterally, indicating an electrical diaschisis, and did not recover
Traversa et al., 1997 [64]	TMS mapping	8 patients with subcortical and 7 patients with cortical lesions		Higher motor threshold, delayed latencies and smaller motor output area in affected hemisphere, increase of output area and clinical improvement after 8 weeks
Cao et al., 1998 [65]	fMRI	8 patients 8/0/0	Hand movements	In 6 patients with extended activation in ipsilateral SM1, in two of them additional ipsilateral activation in premotor and dorsolateral prefrontal cortex
Liepert et al., 1998 [66]	TMS mapping	6 patients in the chronic stage after stroke (3 cortical and 3 subcortical lesions), studied before and after intense physiotherapy (CIMT)		Significant enlargement of motor output area in the affected hemisphere after therapy, shift of the amplitude-weighted center of gravity in affected hemisphere and significant improvement of motor functions
Rossini et al., 1998 [67]	MEG	27 patients		Extension of the sensory hand area in the affected hemisphere and, to a lesser extent, in the unaffected hemisphere
Rossini et al., 1998 [68]	fMRI, MEG, TMS mapping	1 patient with cortical lesion, good recovery		All 3 techniques show an enlargement and posterior shift of SM1 in the affected hemisphere
Seitz et al., 1998 [69]	PET	7 patients with cortical lesions 7/0/0	Active finger movements	Bilateral activation in dorsolateral and medial premotor areas during movement of the affected hand
Silvestrini et al., 1998 [70]	TCD	9 patients 9/0/0	Thumb-to-finger opposition	Stronger increase in flow velocity in the hemisphere ipsilateral to the affected hand. Same result 2–4 months later
Byrnes et al., 1999 [71]	TMS mapping	20 patients with subcortical infarction		Higher motor threshold in affected hemisphere, mediolateral shifts of cortical motor maps especially in longer standing cases
Cuadrado et al., 1999 [72]	TCD	30 patients, studied 1 week, 1 month, and 6 months after stroke	Thumb-to-finger opposition	Strong increase of blood flow velocity in the ipsilateral, healthy hemisphere during movements with the paretic hand. Low blood flow increases in the damaged hemisphere early after stroke, but stronger 6 months later

Author	Technique	Patients and recovery: good/partially/poor	Task	Results
Forss et al., 1999 [73]	SEP	6 patients with parietal lesions		Primary (S1) and secondary (S2) somatosensory cortex may be activated sequentially, S2 ipsilateral to stimulation may receive direct input from the periphery
Green et al., 1999 [74]	EEG	10 patients	Finger movements	In 5 patients, the nonlesioned hemisphere was activated, in 1 patient, a posterior displacement of the motor potential in the affected hemisphere occurred
Kopp et al., 1999 [75]	EEG	3 patients with cortical and 1 patient with subcortical lesion, studied before and after therapy	Finger flexion (1 Hz)	Improvement of motor function after the training; pretreatment: MP in the affected hemisphere more anterior; post-treatment: MP even more anterior and deeper; 3 months later: MP shifted to the nonlesioned hemisphere
Muellbacher et al., 1999 [76]	TMS	6 hemiparetic patients with initial paresis of lingual muscles, good recovery		In controls, ipsi- and contralateral TMS produced motor evoked potentials in lingual muscles; in patients, only TMS of the nonlesioned hemisphere produced lingual MEPs
Nelles et al., 1999 [45]	PET	6 patients with subcortical infarction 0/0/6	Passive arm movements	Stronger activation (compared to controls); bilateral SM1 and inferior parietal cortex, contralateral superior parietal and ipsilateral precuneus
Nelles et al., 1999 [77]	PET	6 patients with subcortical lesions, studied twice within 12 weeks after stroke	Passive arm movements	PET1: bilateral inferior parietal cortex, contralateral SM1, ipsilateral DLPC, SMA and cingulated. PET2: contralateral SM1, bilateral inferior parietal cortex, ipsilateral premotor area, partial clinical recovery from PET1 to PET2
Seitz et al., 1999 [78]	PET	7 patients with cortical infarctions 7/0/0	Finger and hand movements	Lesion-affected network (during resting state): perilesional areas, contralesional motor, medial parietal, lateral occipital cortex, bilateral basal ganglia, and thalamus. Recovery-related network: bilateral occipital and prefrontal areas, contralesional cingulate, hippocampus, dorsal thalamus, bilateral cerebellum. Overlap of both networks in contralesional lateral thalamus, cuneus, bilateral extrastriate cortex
Cramer et al., 2000 [79]	fMRI	1 patient (P1) with infarct in M1, 1 patient (P2) with lesion in S1	Finger tapping and tactile stimulation	P1: finger tapping activated only S1 area P2: tactile stimulation activated only M1
Liepert et al., 2000 [80]	TMS mapping	13 chronic patients (10 subcortical, 3 cortical lesions), tested twice before and 3 times after intensive physiotherapy		Improvement of motor performance after therapy, which persisted for the follow-up of 6 months. Therapy-induced enlargement of cortical motor output area in affected hemisphere and recruitment of adjacent brain areas. Follow-up data indicate an increase of synaptic efficiency in affected hemisphere
Liepert et al., 2000 [81]	TMS mapping	9 subacute stroke patients, tested before and after a single 1.5 h session of physiotherapy		After therapy, dexterity of the paretic hand was improved and motor output area in the affected hemisphere was enlarged. This effect was partially reversed 1 day later

Table 1. Imaging studies of motor and somatosensory areas after stroke (continued).

Author	Technique	Patients and recovery: good/partially/poor	Task	Results
Marshall et al., 2000 [82]	fMRI	6 patients with lacunar lesions, studied early and 3–6 months after stroke	Finger-thumb-opposition	Patients showed greater activations in ipsilateral SM cortex, ipsilateral posterior parietal and bilateral prefrontal areas. Improvement of motor functions was associated with stronger activation in the contralateral SM cortex
Wikstrom et al., 2000 [83]	MEG	14 patients studied twice: 14 days and 3 months after stroke		At follow-up, P1 amplitude was increased in 6 patients, which was correlated with an improvement of two-point discrimination ability
Binkowski et al., 2001 [39]	MRI	52 patients		Initial motor score but not lesion size was correlated with outcome
Calautti et al., 2001 [84]	PET	5 patients, striatocapsular lesion, studied 7 (PET 1) and 31 (PET 2) weeks after stroke	Thumb-to-index tapping	At PET 1: strong bilateral activations. At PET 2: less activity in both hemispheres, but new activations in prefrontal and premotor area and putamen in the unaffected hemisphere
Calautti et al., 2001 [85]	PET	5 patients with subcortical stroke, studied twice over months	Thumb-to-index tapping	Hemispheric activation shifted towards the unaffected hemisphere in patients with poorer recovery
Levy et al., 2001 [86]	fMRI	1 stroke patient, studied before and after CIMT	Sequential finger tapping	Prior to CIMT: activity in contralesional parietal and occipital cortex; after CIMT: activations bordering the lesion, bilateral association motor cortex activations, contralesional M1 activation
Liepert et al., 2001 [87]	TMS mapping	9 patients, 1 week of conventional physiotherapy compared with 1 week of forced use therapy		Enlargement of motor output area of paretic hand muscle and improvement of motor function only after forced use therapy. Significantly stronger cog. shifts in the affected hemisphere
Nelles et al., 2001 [88]	PET	10 patients before and after arm training	Passive hand movements	Before treatment: bilateral activations in inferior parietal cortex. After treatment: additional activations in bilateral premotor cortex and contralateral SMA
Pariente et al., 2001 [89]	fMRI	Placebo-controlled study of 8 patients with lacunar stroke, single dose of fluoxetine	Active and passive hand movements	Fluoxetine improved motor skills and enhanced activity in the ipsilesional primary motor cortex
Pineiro et al., 2001 [90]	fMRI	8 patients with subcortical infarcts, compared with 20 healthy controls	Sequential finger tapping	Patients had a decreased motor cortex lateralization index; activity was shifted posteriorly in the lesioned hemisphere

Author	Technique	Patients and recovery: good/partially/poor	Task	Results
Rossini et al., 2001 [91]	MEG/MRI	17 chronic stroke patients		Asymmetry between the two hemispheres, enlargements of hand area and dipole strength in affected hemisphere particularly after cortical lesions
Staines et al., 2001 [92]	fMRI	2 patients, tested 3 times during recovery	Gripping task	Initially, bilateral movements enhanced activity in M1 of the affected hemisphere stronger than unilateral paretic hand movements. Difference disappeared with recovery
Watanabe et al., 2001 [93]	MRI	DTI of corticospinal tracts in 16 patients		DTI allowed detection of Wallerian degeneration 2-3 weeks after stroke
Carey et al., 2002 [94]	fMRI	10 chronic stroke patients studied before and after a finger movement tracking program	Tracking task	Pretreatment: activation mainly in unaffected hemisphere; post-treatment: activation mainly in affected hemisphere, accompanied by improved motor performance
Feydy et al., 2002 [95]	fMRI	Longitudinal study of 14 patients 1 to 6 months after stroke		2 patterns of activation were found: persisting activation in unaffected hemisphere in patients with lesioned M1, patients without M1 lesion develop activity mainly in affected hemisphere
Kato et al., 2002 [96]	fMRI/NIRS	6 stroke patients, comparison of fMRI and NIRS results	Hand movements	Paretic hand movements activated both M1 areas. NIRS had lower spatial resolution but provided a dynamic profile of activation.
Small et al., 2002 [97]	fMRI	Longitudinal study of 12 patients: 6 with good, 6 with poor recovery	Finger and wrist movements	Changes of activity in the cerebellum opposite the injured corticospinal tract correlated with recovery

Table 1. Imaging studies of motor and somatosensory areas after stroke (continued).
CIMT: constraint induced movement therapy; DTI: Diffusion tensor imaging; DLPC: dorsolateral prefrontal cortex; EEG: electroencephalogram; fMRI: functional magnetic resonance imaging; M1: primary motor cortex; MEG: magnetoencephalography; MEP: motor evoked potential; MP: motor potential; MRI: magnetic resonance imaging; MRP: movement related potential; NIRS: near-infrared spectroscopy; PET: positron emission tomography; rCBF: relative cerebral blood flow; S1: primary somatosensory cortex; S2: secondary somatosensory cortex; SEP: somatosensory evoked potential; SM1: primary sensorimotor cortex; SMA: supplementary motor area; SPECT: single photon emission computed tomography; TCD: transcranial Doppler ultrasonography; TMS: transcranial magnetic stimulation.

Recovery and plasticity imaging in stroke patients

Author	Technique	Patients and recovery: good/partially/poor	Task	Results
Soh et al., 1978 [124]	Xenon 133	13 patients with left cortical lesions	Simple speech test	Motor aphasia: evidence of cortical dysfunction in lower part of rolandic area, less consistent in Broca's area. Sensory aphasia: dysfunction in superior-posterior temporal cortex
Walker-Batson et al., 1988 [125]	SPECT	1 patient with crossed aphasia due to right cortical lesion	Phoneme detection test; mathematical test	Phoneme detection: activation in both frontal lobes. Mathematical test: activation in both right temporal and parietal lobes
Karbe et al., 1990 [126]	PET (glucose)	26 patients (12 with cortical lesions; 7 with cortical and subcortical lesions; 7 with subcortical lesions		Reduced glucose metabolism in left convexity cortex and left basal ganglia. Results of Aachener Aphasie Test were correlated with left parietotemporal metabolism
Metter, 1991 [127]	PET (glucose)			Metabolic abnormalities in left temporoparietal region in all patients; additional metabolic changes in structurally undamaged areas: left prefrontal lobe, basal ganglia, and thalamus
Heiss et al., 1993 [128]	PET (glucose)	26 patients, 17 were tested twice		The increase in metabolism in the left hemisphere was correlated with the recovery from aphasia
Mlcoch et al., 1994 [129]	SPECT	14 patients with Broca's aphasia, tested within 1 month and 3 months after infarction		Initial hypoperfusion of basal ganglia, periventricular white matter, and inferior frontal areas. rCBF in inferior frontal area was associated with recovery of fluent speech
Engelien et al., 1995 [130]	PET (H₂O)	1 patient with auditory agnosia	Passive listening and sound categorization	After recovery, the patient activated a bihemispherical network comprising frontal, middle temporal, and inferior parietal cortices, right cerebellum, right caudate nucleus, left anterior cingulate gyrus
Karbe et al., 1995 [131]	PET (glucose)	22 patients with left cortical infarction		Word fluency correlated with metabolism in left prefrontal cortex. Receptive language disorder correlated with metabolism in left superior temporal cortex
Weiller et al., 1995 [132]	PET (H₂O)	6 patients recovered from Wernicke's aphasia	Repetition of pseudowords; verb generation task	rCBF increases in bilateral frontal areas, right hemispheric superior temporal gyrus, and inferior premotor area
Belin et al., 1996 [133]	PET (H₂O)	7 patients with Broca's aphasia	Repetition of simple words; repetition of words trained during melodic intonation therapy (MIT)	Simple words: activation of right hemispheric language areas and deactivation of homotopic left hemispheric areas. MIT-associated words: activation of left Broca's area and left prefrontal cortex, and deactivation of right parietotemporal areas

Table 2. Language imaging studies after stroke.

Author	Technique	Patients and recovery: good/partially/poor	Task	Results
Ohyama et al., 1996 [134]	PET (H$_2$O)	16 patients (10 with Wernicke's aphasia, 6 with Broca's aphasia)	Word repetition task	Compared to controls, the patients had stronger activations in right hemispheric posteroinferofrontal and posterosuperotemporal areas
Cappa et al., 1997 [135]	PET (glucose)	8 patients, tested twice: within 2 weeks and 6 months after stroke	Word repetition task	Initial hypometabolism in both hemispheres: improvement of language function correlated with increased glucose metabolism in right hemispheric regions
Heiss et al., 1997 [136]	PET (glucose)	6 patients, tested twice: 4 weeks and 12–18 months after stroke	Word repetition task	Clinical improvement (observed in 3 patients) was related to left hemispheric speech areas, especially left superior temporal gyrus. Poor outcome (3 patients) was associated with increased metabolism in right hemispheric regions
Thomas et al., 1997 [137]	EEG (DC recordings)	11 patients, tested during aphasia and after recovery	Single word processing	During aphasia: DC negativity was bilateral (while in controls it has a left frontal maximum). After recovery: patients with Broca's aphasia showed a left frontal lateralization; in Wernicke's aphasia the DC negativity shifted further to the right hemisphere
Karbe et al., 1998 [138]	PET (glucose)		Word repetition task	In the subacute stage after stroke, left SMA showed enhanced activation. Long-term prognosis was associated with restitution of the left superior temporal cortex. Right hemispheric regions were activated when homologous areas remained impaired. However, this strategy was less effective
Mimura et al., 1998 [139]	SPECT	Prospective study: 20 patients with left hemispheric lesions, studied twice: 3 and 9 months post stroke. Retrospective study: 16 aphasic patients, studied 83 months post-onset		Prospective study: initial language deficit was correlated with initial rCBF in left hemisphere. At follow-up: left hemispheric rCBF change was correlated with improvement of aphasia. Retrospective study: good recovery of language function was associated with increased rCBF in right hemispheric frontal and thalamic regions and left frontal region
Muller et al., 1998 [140]	PET (H$_2$O)	12 children with left hemispheric, and 9 children with right hemispheric lesions	Listening and repetition	Left hemispheric lesioned children predominantly had a shift of activations into the right hemisphere. Right hemispheric lesioned children showed activations in subcortical and cerebellar areas
Small et al., 1998 [141]	fMRI	1 patient with dyslexia, studied before and after linguistic therapy	Reading task	Prior to therapy, the patient was unable to read 'nonwords'. Posttreatment, the patient was able to read nonwords and function words and had adopted a new reading technique. Brain activation during reading was pretreatment in left angular gyrus, and posttherapy in left lingual gyrus.

Author	Technique	Patients and recovery: good/partially/poor	Task	Results
Cao et al., 1999 [142]	fMRI	7 aphasic patients with good recovery, tested 38 months (range: 5–144) after stroke	Picture naming task; word generation task	Compared to healthy volunteers, patients had increased activation in the right hemisphere. In patients, bihemispheric activations were associated with a better language outcome than only right hemispheric activations.
Heiss et al., 1999 [143]	PET (H_2O)	23 aphasic patients, studied 2 and 8 weeks after stroke (7 frontal, 7 temporal, 9 subcortical lesions)	Word repetition task	Patients with subcortical and frontal lesions improved substantially. Initially, they had activations in right inferior frontal and right superior temporal gyri. At follow-up, they activated the left superior temporal gyrus. Patients with temporal lesions improved only in word comprehension. At baseline, they activated left Broca's area and the right superior temporal gyrus. At follow-up, they activated the precentral gyrus bilaterally and the right superior temporal gyrus
Miura et al., 1999 [144]	fMRI	1 patient with Broca's aphasia	Verbal tasks	Recovery of language function was associated with an increment of activation in the left frontal lobe
Musso et al., 1999 [145]	PET (H_2O)	4 patients with Wernicke's aphasia, studied before and after each of 11 language comprehension training sessions	Language comprehension task	Training-induced improvement of verbal comprehension in all patients. These improvements correlated with activations in the posterior part of the right superior temporal gyrus and in the left precuneus
Thulborn et al., 1999 [146]	fMRI	1 patient with Broca's aphasia (stroke), 1 patient with Wernicke's aphasia (neurosurgery)	Word comprehension	Shifts of activation to homologous brain areas in the right hemisphere, paralleled by improvement of language
Warburton et al., 1999 [147]	PET (H_2O)	6 aphasic patients	Word retrieval task	In controls and patients, the task induced a left lateralized inferolateral temporal activation and a right prefrontal involvement in ~50%
Calvert et al., 2000 [148]	fMRI	1 patient with left frontal lesion	Verbal semantic decision task and rhyme judgement	Verbal semantic decision task: no activation of Broca's area (in contrast to controls). Rhyme judgement: activation in Broca's area, much stronger in right than left (perilesional) hemisphere
Gold and Kertesz, 2000 [149]	fMRI	1 patient, large damage to left-hemisphere language structures	Semantic processing of visual words	Activation of right-hemispheric perisylvian and extrasylvian temporal regions

Table 2. Language imaging studies after stroke (continued).

DC: direct current; EEG: electroencephalogram; fMRI: functional magnetic resonance imaging; MIT: melodic intonation therapy; PET: positron emission tomography; rCBF: relative cerebral blood flow; SMA: supplementary motor area; SPECT: single photon emission computed tomography.

References

1.   Merzenich MM, Kaas JH, Wall JT et al. Topographic reorganization of somatosensory cortical areas 3b and 1 in adult monkeys following restricted deafferentation. *Neuroscience* 1983;8:33–55.

2.   Merzenich MM, Kaas JH, Wall JT et al. Progression of change following median nerve section in the cortical representation of the hand in areas 3b and 1 in adult owl and squirrel monkeys. *Neuroscience* 1983;10:639–65.

3.   Merzenich MM, Nelson RJ, Stryker MP et al. Somatosensory cortical map changes following digit amputation in adult monkeys. *J Comp Neurol.* 1984;224:591–605.

4.   Nudo RJ, Milliken GW. Reorganisation of movement representations in primary motor cortex following focal ischemic infarcts in adult squirrel monkeys. *J Neurophysiol* 1996;75:2144–9.

5.   Pons TP, Garraghty PE, Ommaya AK et al. Massive cortical reorganization after sensory deafferentation in adult macaques. *Science* 1991;252:1857–60.

6.   Sanes JN, Suner S, Lando JF et al. Rapid reorganization of adult rat motor cortex somatic representation patterns after motor nerve injury. *Proc Natl Acad Sci USA* 1988;85:2003–7.

7.   Sanes JN, Wang J, Donoghue JP. Immediate and delayed changes of rat motor cortical output representation with new forelimb configurations. *Cereb Cortex* 1992;2:141–52.

8.   Castro-Alamancos MA, Borrell J. Functional recovery of forelimb response capacity after forelimb primary motor cortex damage in the rat is due to the reorganization of adjacent areas of cortex. *Neuroscience* 1995;68:793–805.

9.   Rouiller EM, Yu XH, Moret V et al. Dexterity in adult monkeys following early lesion of the motor cortical hand area: the role of cortex adjacent to the lesion. *Eur J Neurosci* 1998;10:729–40.

10. Liu Y, Rouiller EM. Mechanisms of recovery of dexterity following unilateral lesion of the sensorimotor cortex in adult monkeys. *Exp Brain Res* 1999;128:149–59.

11. Nudo RJ, Milliken GW, Jenkins WM et al. Use-dependent alterations of movement representations in primary motor cortex of adult squirrel monkeys. *J Neurosci* 1996;16:785–807.

12. Nudo RJ, Wise BM, SiFuentes F et al. Neural substrates for the effects of rehabilitative training on motor recovery after ischemic infarct. *Science* 1996;272:1791–4.

13. Schallert T, Kozlowski DA, Humm JL et al. Use-dependent structural events in recovery of function. *Adv Neurol* 1997;73:229–38.

14. Florence SL, Taub HB, Kaas JH. Large-scale sprouting of cortical connections after peripheral injury in adult macaque monkeys. *Science* 1998;282:1117–21.

15. Xerri C, Merzenich MM, Peterson BE et al. Plasticity of primary somatosensory cortex paralleling sensorimotor skill recovery from stroke in adult monkeys. *J Neurophysiol* 1998;79:2119–48.

16. Florence SL, Kaas JH. Large-scale reorganization at multiple levels of the somatosensory pathway follows therapeutic amputation of the hand in monkeys. *J Neurosci* 1995;15:8083–95.

17. Jones EG, Pons T. Thalamic and brain stem contributions to large-scale plasticity of primate somatosensory cortex. *Science* 1998;282:1121–5.

18. Woods TM, Cusick CG, Pons TP et al. Progressive transneuronal changes in the brainstem and thalamus after long-term dorsal rhizotomies in adult macaque monkeys. *J Neurosci* 2000;20(10):3884–99.

19. Garraghty PE, Muja N. NMDA receptors and plasticity in adult primate somatosensory cortex. *J Comp Neurol* 1996;367:319–26.

20. Hess G, Donoghue JP. Long-term potentiation of horizontal connections provides a mechanism to reorganize cortical motor maps. *J Neurophysiol* 1994;71:2543–7.

21. Kano M, Iino K, Kano M. Functional reorganization of adult cat somatosensory cortex is dependent on NMDA receptors. *Neuroreport* 1991;2:77–80.

22. Que M, Schiene K, Witte OW et al. Widespread up-regulation of N-methyl-D-aspartate receptors after focal photothrombotic lesion in rat brain. *Neurosci Lett* 1999;273:77–80.

23. Jacobs KM, Donoghue JP. Reshaping the cortical motor map by unmasking latent intracortical connections. *Science* 1991;251:944–7.

24. Hess G, Aizenman CD, Donoghue JP. Conditions for the induction of long-term potentiation in layer II/III horizontal connections of the rat motor cortex. *J Neurophysiol* 1996;75:1765–78.

25. Hess G, Donoghue JP. Long-term potentiation and long-term depression of horizontal connections in rat motor cortex. *Acta Neurobiol Exp* 1996;56:397–405.

26. Hess G, Donoghue JP. Long-term depression of horizontal connections in rat motor cortex. *Eur J Neurosci* 1996;8:658–65.

27. Jones EG. GABAergic neurons and their role in cortical plasticity in primates. *Cereb Cortex* 1993;3:361–72.

28. Neumann-Haefelin T, Staiger JF, Redecker C et al. Immunohistochemical evidence for dysregulation of the GABAergic system ipsilateral to photochemically induced cortical infarcts in rats. *Neuroscience* 1998;87:871–9.

29. Que M, Witte OW, Neumann-Haefelin T et al. Changes in GABA(A) and GABA(B) receptor binding following cortical photothrombosis: a quantitative receptor autoradiographic study. *Neuroscience* 1999;93:1233–40.

30. Kilgard MP, Merzenich MM. Cortical map reorganization enabled by nucleus basalis activity. *Science* 1998;279:1714–8.

31. Kirkwood A, Rozas C, Kirkwood J et al. Modulation of long-term synaptic depression in visual cortex by acetylcholine and norepinephrine. *J Neurosci* 1999;19:1599–609.

32. Oyesiku NM, Evans CO, Houston S et al. Regional changes in the expression of neurotrophic factors and their receptors following acute traumatic brain injury in the adult rat brain. *Brain Res* 1999;833:161–72.

33. Kokaia Z, Andsberg G, Yan Q et al. Rapid alterations of BDNF protein levels in the rat brain after focal ischemia: evidence for increased synthesis and anterograde axonal transport. *Exp Neurol* 1998;154:289–301.

34. Hughes PE, Alexi T, Walton M et al. Activity and injury-dependent expression of inducible transcription factors, growth factors and apoptosis-related genes within the central nervous system. *Prog Neurobiol* 1999;57:421–50.

35. Jones TA, Schallert T. Overgrowth and pruning of dendrites in adult rats recovering from neocortial damage. *Brain Res* 1992;581:156–60.

36. Jones TA, Schallert T. Use-dependent growth of pyramidal neurons after neocortical damage. *J Neurosci* 1994;14:2140–52.

37. Jones TA, Kleim JA, Greenough WT. Synaptogenesis and dendritic growth in the cortex opposite unilateral sensorimotor cortex damage in adult rats: a quantitative electron microscopic examination. *Brain Res* 1996;733:142–8.

38. Johansson BB. Brain plasticity and stroke rehabilitation. *Stroke* 2000;31:223–30.

39. Binkofski F, Seitz RJ, Hacklander T et al. Recovery of motor functions following hemiparetic stroke: a clinical and magnetic resonance-morphometric study. *Cerebrovasc Dis* 2001;11:273–81.

40. Cohen LG, Ziemann U, Chen R et al. Studies of neuroplasticity with transcranial magnetic stimulation. *J Clin Neurophysiol* 1998;15(4):305–24.

41. Von Monakow C. Lokalisation im Gehirn und funktionelle Störungen induziert durch kortikale Läsionen. Wiesbaden, Germany: Bergmann JF, 1914.

42. Kujirai T, Caramia MD, Rothwell JC et al. Corticocortical inhibition in human motor cortex. *J Physiol* 1993;471:501–19.

43. Cohen LG, Celnik P, Pascual-Leone A et al. Functional relevance of cross-modal plasticity in blind humans. *Nature* 1997;389:180–3.

44. Weiller C, Chollet F, Friston KJ et al. Functional reorganization of the brain in recovery from striatocapsular infarction in man. *Ann Neurol* 1992;31:463–72.

45. Nelles G, Spiekermann G, Jueptner M et al. Reorganization of sensory and motor systems in hemiplegic stroke patients. A positron emission tomography study. *Stroke* 1999;30:1510–6.

46. Rijntjes M, Tegenthoff M, Liepert J et al. Cortical reorganization in patients with facial palsy. *Ann Neurol* 1997;41:621–30.

47. Liepert J, Oreja-Guevara C, Cohen LG et al. Plasticity of cortical hand muscle representation in patients with hemifacial spasm. *Neurosci Lett* 1999;272:33–36.

48. Flor H, Elbert T, Knecht S et al. Phantom-limb pain as a perceptual correlate of cortical reorganization following arm amputation. *Nature* 1995;375:482–4.

49. Birbaumer N, Lutzenberger W, Montoya P et al. Effects of regional anesthesia on phantom limb pain are mirrored in changes in cortical reorganization. *J Neurosci* 1997;17:5503–8.

50. Robertson ICH. Cognitive rehabilitation: attention and neglect. *Trends Cogn Sci* 1999;3(10):385–93.

51. Weiller C. Imaging recovery from stroke. *Exp Brain Res* 1998;123:13–7.

52. Chollet F, DiPiero V, Wise RJ et al. The functional anatomy of motor recovery after stroke in humans: a study with positron emission tomography. *Ann Neurol* 1991;29(1):63–71.

53. Weiller C, Ramsay SC, Wise RJS et al. Individual patterns of functional reorganization in the human cerebral cortex after capsular infarction. *Ann Neurol* 1993;33:181–89.

54. Weder B, Knorr U, Herzog H et al. Tactile exploration of shape after subcortical ischaemic infarction studied with PET. *Brain* 1994;117(3):593–605.

55. Weder B, Seitz RJ. Deficient cerebral activation pattern in stroke recovery. *Neuroreport* 1994;5(4):457–60.

56. Binkofski F, Seitz RJ, Arnold S et al. Thalamic metabolism and corticospinal tract integrity determine motor recovery in stroke. *Ann Neurol* 1996;39(4):460–70.

57. Iglesias S, Marchal G, Rioux P et al. Do changes in oxygen metabolism in the affected cerebral hemisphere underlie early neurological recovery after stroke? A positron emission tomography study. *Stroke* 1996;27(7):1192–9.

58. Pantano P, Formisano R, Ricci M et al. Motor recovery after stroke. Morphological and functional brain alterations. *Brain* 1996;119:1849–57.

59. Cicinelli P, Traversa R, Rossini PM. Post-stroke reorganization of brain motor output to the hand: a 2-4 month follow-up with focal magnetic transcranial stimulation. *Electroencephalogr Clin Neurophysiol* 1997;105:438–50.

60. Cramer SC, Nelles G, Benson RR et al. A functional MRI study of subjects recovered from hemiparetic stroke. *Stroke* 1997;28:2518–27.

61. Dettmers C, Stephan KM, Lemon RN et al. Reorganization of the executive motor system after stroke. *Cerebrovasc Dis* 1997;7:187–200.

62. Honda M, Nagamine T, Fukuyama H et al. Movement-related cortical potentials and regional cerebral blood flow change in patients with stroke after motor recovery. *J Neurol Sci* 1997;146(2):117–26.

63. Juhasz C, Kamondi A, Szirmai I. Spectral EEG analysis following hemispheric stroke: evidences of transhemispheric diaschisis. *Acta Neurol Scand* 1997;96(6):397–400.

64. Traversa R, Cicinelli P, Bassi A et al. Mapping of motor cortical reorganization after stroke. A brain stimulation study with focal magnetic pulses. *Stroke* 1997;28:110–7.

65. Cao Y, D´Olhaberriague L, Vikingstad EM et al. Pilot study of functional MRI to assess cerebral activation of motor function after poststroke hemiparesis. *Stroke* 1998;29(1):112–22.

66. Liepert J, Miltner WHR, Bauder H et al. Motor cortex plasticity during constraint–induced movement therapy in stroke patients. *Neurosci Lett* 1998;250:5–8.

67. Rossini PM, Caltagirone C, Castriota-Scanderbeg A et al. Hand motor cortical area reorganization in stroke: a study with fMRI, MEG and TCS maps. *NeuroReport* 1998;9:2141–6.

68. Rossini PM, Tecchio F, Pizzella V et al. On the reorganization of sensory hand areas after mono-hemispheric lesion: a functional (MEG)/anatomical (MRI) integrative study. *Brain Res* 1998;782(1–2):153–66.

69. Seitz RJ, Hoflich P, Binkofski F et al. Role of the premotor cortex in recovery from middle cerebral artery infarction. *Arch Neurol* 1998;55(8):1081–8.

70. Silvestrini M, Cupini LM, Placidi F et al. Bilateral hemispheric activation in the early recovery of motor function after stroke. *Stroke* 1998;29(7):1305–10.

71. Byrnes ML, Thickbroom GW, Phillips BA et al. Physiological studies of the corticomotor projection to the hand after subcortical stroke. *Clin Neurophysiol* 1999;110:487–98.

72. Cuadrado ML, Egido JA, Gonzalez-Gutierrez JL et al. Bihemispheric contribution to motor recovery after stroke: A longitudinal study with transcranial doppler ultrasonography. *Cerebrovasc Dis* 1999;9(6):337–44.

73. Forss N, Hietanen M, Salonen O et al. Modified activation of somatosensory cortical network in patients with right–hemisphere stroke. *Brain* 1999;122(Pt 10):1889–99.

74. Green JB, Bialy Y, Sora E et al. High-resolution EEG in poststroke hemiparesis can identify ipsilateral generators during motor tasks. *Stroke* 1999;30(12):2659–65.

75. Kopp B, Kunkel A, Muehlnickel W et al. Plasticity in the motor system related to therapy-induced improvement of movement after stroke. *Neuroreport* 1998;10:807–10.

76. Muellbacher W, Artner C, Mamoli B. The role of the intact hemisphere in recovery of midline muscles after recent monohemispheric stroke. *J Neurol* 1999;246:250–6.

77. Nelles G, Spiekermann G, Jueptner M et al. Evolution of functional reorganization in hemiplegic stroke: a serial positron emission tomographic activation study. *Ann Neurol* 1999;46:901–9.

78. Seitz RJ, Azari NP, Knorr U et al. The role of diaschisis in stroke recovery. *Stroke* 1999;30:1844–50.

79. Cramer SC, Moore CI, Finklestein SP et al. A pilot study of somatotopic mapping after cortical infarct. *Stroke* 2000;31:668–71.

80. Liepert J, Bauder H, Miltner WHR et al. Treatment-induced cortical reorganization after stroke in humans. *Stroke* 2000;31:1210–6.

81. Liepert J, Graef S, Uhde I et al. Training-induced changes of motor cortex representations in stroke patients. *Acta Neurol Scand* 2000;101:321–6.

82. Marshall RS, Perera GM, Lazar RM et al. Evolution of cortical activation during recovery from corticospinal tract infarction. *Stroke* 2000;31(3):656–61.

83. Wikström H, Roine RO, Aronen HJ et al. Specific changes in somatosensory evoked magnetic fields during recovery from sensorimotor stroke. *Ann Neurol* 2000;47:353–60.

84. Calautti C, Leroy F, Guincestre JY et al. Dynamics of motor network overactivation after striatocapsular stroke: a longitudinal PET study using a fixed-performance paradigm. *Stroke* 2001;32:2534–42.

85. Calautti C, Leroy F, Guincestre JY et al. Sequential activation brain mapping after subcortical stroke: changes in hemispheric balance and recovery. *Neuroreport* 2001;12:3883–6.

86. Levy CE, Nichols DS, Schmalbrock PM et al. Functional MRI evidence of cortical reorganization in upper–limb stroke hemiplegia treated with constraint-induced movement therapy. *Am J Phys Med Rehabil* 2001;80:4–12.

87. Liepert J, Uhde I, Gräf S et al. Motor cortex plasticity during forced use therapy in stroke patients. *J Neurol* 2001;248:315–21.

88. Nelles G, Jentzen W, Jueptner M et al. Arm training induced brain plasticity in stroke studied with serial positron emission tomography. *Neuroimage* 2001;13:1146–54.

89. Pariente J, Loubinoux I, Carel C et al. Fluoxetine modulates motor performance and cerebral activation of patients recovering from stroke. *Ann Neurol* 2001;50:718–29.

90. Pineiro R, Pendlebury S, Johansen-Berg H, et al. Functional MRI detects posterior shifts in primary sensorimotor cortex activation after stroke: evidence of local adaptive reorganization? *Stroke* 2001;32:1134–9.

91. Rossini PM, Tecchio F, Pizzella V et al. Interhemispheric differences of sensory hand areas after monohemispheric stroke: MEG/MRI integrative study. *Neuroimage* 2001;142:474–85.

92. Staines WR, McIlroy WE, Graham SJ et al. Bilateral movement enhances ipsilesional cortical activity in acute stroke: a pilot functional MRI study. *Neurology* 2001;56:401–4.

93. Watanabe T, Honda Y, Fujii Y, et al. Three-dimensional anisotropy contrast magnetic resonance axonography to predict the prognosis for motor function in patients suffering from stroke. *J Neurosurg* 2001;94:955–60.

94. Carey JR, Kimberley TJ, Lewis SM et al. Analysis of fMRI and finger tracking training in subjects with chronic stroke. *Brain* 2002;125:773–88.

95. Feydy A, Carlier R, Roby-Brami A, et al. Longitudinal study of motor recovery after stroke: recruitment and focusing of brain activation. *Stroke* 2002;33:1610–7.

96. Kato H, Izumiyama M, Koizumi H et al. Near-infrared spectroscopic topography as a tool to monitor motor reorganization after hemiparetic stroke: a comparison with functional MRI. *Stroke* 2002;33:2032–6.

97. Small SL, Hlustik P, Noll DC et al. Cerebellar hemispheric activation ipsilateral to the paretic hand correlates with functional recovery after stroke. *Brain* 2002;125:1544–57.

98. Rizzolatti G, Luppino G, Matelli M. The organization of the cortical motor system: new concepts. *Electroencephalogr Clin Neurophysiol* 1998;106:283–96.

99. Weiller C, Rijntjes M. Learning, plasticity, and recovery in the central nervous system. *Exp Brain Res* 1999;128:134–8.

100. Hutchins KD, Martino AM, Strick PL. Corticospinal projections from the medial wall of the hemisphere. *Exp Brain Res* 1988;71:667–72.

101. Dum RP, Strick PL. The origin of corticospinal projections from the premotor areas in the frontal lobe. *J Neurosci* 1991;11:667–89.

102. Price CJ, Wise RJ, Watson JD et al. Brain activation during reading. The effects of exposure duration and task. *Brain* 1994;117:1255–69.

103. Witte OW. Lesion-induced plasticity as a potential mechanism for recovery and rehabilitative training. *Curr Opin Neurol* 1998;11:655–62.

104. Liepert J, Storch P, Fritsch A et al. Motor cortex disinhibition in acute stroke. *Clin Neurophysiol* 2000;111:671–6.

105. Liepert J, Hamzei F, Weiller C. Motor cortex disinhibition of the unaffected hemisphere after acute stroke *Muscle Nerve* 2000;23:1761–3.

106. Shimizu T, Hosaki A, Hino T et al. Motor cortical disinhibition in the unaffected hemisphere after unilateral cortical stroke. *Brain* 2002;125:1896–1907.

107. Caramia MD, Iani C, Bernardi G. Cerebral plasticity after stroke as revealed by ipsilateral responses to magnetic stimulation. *Neuroreport* 1996;7:1756–60.

108. Netz J, Lammers T, Hömberg V. Reorganization of motor output in the non-affected hemisphere after stroke. *Brain* 1997,120:1579–86.

109. Turton A, Wroe S, Trepte N et al. Contralateral and ipsilateral EMG responses to transcranial magnetic stimulation during recovery of arm and hand function after stroke. *Electroencephalogr Clin Neurophysiol* 1996;101:316–28.

110. Palmer E, Ashby P, Hajek VE. Ipsilateral fast corticospinal pathways do not account for recovery in stroke. *Ann Neurol* 1992;32(4):519–25.

111. Hamdy S, Aziz Q, Rothwell JC et al. Recovery of swallowing after dysphagic stroke relates to functional reorganization in the intact motor cortex. *Gastroenterology* 1998;115(5):1104–12.

112. Pascual-Leone A, Walsh V, Rothwell J. Transcranial magnetic stimulation in cognitive neuroscience–virtual lesion, chronometry, and functional connectivity. *Curr Opin Neurobiol* 2000;10(2):232–7.

113. Walsh V, Ashbridge E, Cowey A. Cortical plasticity in perceptual learning demonstrated by transcranial magnetic stimulation. *Neuropsychologia* 1998;36(4):363–7.

114. Walsh V, Ellison A, Battelli L et al. Task-specific impairments and enhancements induced by magnetic stimulation of human visual area V5. *Proc R Soc Lond B Biol Sci* 1998;265(1395):537–43.

115. Johansen-Berg H, Rushworth MFS, Matthews PM. A TMS study of the functional significance of ipsilateral motor cortical activation after stroke. 8th International conference for Functional Mapping of the Human Brain, June 2–6, 2002, Sendai, Japan. *Neuroimage* 2002.
Available from URL: http://www.apnet.com/www/journal/hbm2002/13746.html#13746

116. Weiller C. Brain representation of active and passive movements. *Neuroimage* 1996;4:105–10.

117. Weiller C, Leonhardt G, Rijntjes M et al. Early sensory reorganization predicts recovery of lost motor function after stroke - a clinical PET study. *Neuroimage* 1997;5:S28.

118. Stephan KM, Fink GR, Passingham RE et al. Functional anatomy of the mental representation of upper extremity movements in healthy subjects. *J Neurophysiol* 1995;73(1):373–86.

119. Johnson SH. Imagining the impossible: intact motor representations in hemiplegics. *Neuroreport* 2000;11:729–32.

120. Vallar G. The anatomical basis of spatial neglect in humans. In: Robertson ICH, Marshall JC, editors. *Unilateral neglect: Clinical and experimental studies*. New York: Erlbaum Inc, 1993:27–59.

121. Vuilleumier P, Hester D, Assal G et al. Unilateral spatial neglect recovery after sequential strokes. *Neurology* 1996;46(1):184–9.

122. Perani D, Vallar G, Paulesu E et al. Left and right hemisphere contribution to recovery from neglect after right hemisphere damage - an[18F]FDG PET study of two cases. *Neuropsychologia* 1993;31(2):115–25.

123. Pizzamiglio L, Perani D, Cappa SF et al. Recovery of neglect after right hemispheric damage: H2(15)O positron emission tomographic activation study. *Arch Neurol* 1998;55(4):561–8.

124. Soh K, Larsen B, Skinhoj E et al. Regional cerebral blood flow in aphasia. *Arch Neurol* 1978;35(1):625–32.

125. Walker-Batson D, Wendt JS, Devous MD Sr et al. A long-term follow-up case study of crossed aphasia assessed by single-photon emission tomography (SPECT), language, and neuropsychological testing. *Brain Lang* 1988;33(2):311–22.

126. Karbe H, Szelies B, Herholz K et al. Impairment of language is related to left parieto–temporal glucose metabolism in aphasic stroke patients. *J Neurol* 1990;237(1):19–23.

127. Metter EJ. Brain-behavior relationships in aphasia studied by positron emission tomography. *Ann N Y Acad Sci* 1991;620:153–64.

128. Heiss WD, Kessler J, Karbe H et al. Cerebral glucose metabolism as a predictor of recovery from aphasia in ischemic stroke. *Arch Neurol* 1993;50(9):958–64.

129. Mloch AG, Bushnell DL, Gupta S et al. Speech fluency in aphasia. Regional cerebral blood flow correlates of recovery using single-photon emission computed tomography. *J Neuroimaging* 1994;4(1):6–10.

130. Engelien A, Silbersweig D, Stern E et al. The functional anatomy of recovery from auditory agnosia. A PET study of sound categorization in a neurological patient and normal controls. *Brain* 1995;118(Pt 6):1395–1409.

131. Karbe H, Kessler J, Herholz K et al. Long-term prognosis of post-stroke aphasia studied with positron emission tomography. *Arch Neurol* 1995;52(2):186–90.

132. Weiller C, Isensee C, Rijntjes M et al. Recovery from Wernicke´s aphasia: a positron emission tomographic study. *Ann Neurol* 1995;37(6):723–32.

133. Ohyama M, Senda M, Kitamura S et al. Role of the nondominant hemisphere and undamaged area during word repetition in poststroke aphasics. A PET activation study. *Stroke* 1996;27(5):897–903.

134. Belin P, Van Eeckhout P, Zilbovicius M et al. Recovery from nonfluent aphasia after melodic intonation therapy: a PET study. *Neurology* 1996;47(6):1504–11.

135. Cappa SF, Perani D, Grassi F et al. A PET follow-up study of recovery after stroke in acute aphasics. *Brain Lang* 1997;56(1):55–67.

136. Heiss WD, Karbe H, Weber-Luxenburger G et al. Speech-induced cerebral metabolic activation reflects recovery from aphasia. *J Neurol Sci* 1997;145(2):213–7.

137. Thomas C, Altenmueller E, Marckmann G et al. Language processing in aphasia: changes in lateralization patterns during recovery reflect cerebral plasticity in adults. *Electroencephalogr Clin Neurophysiol* 1997;102(2):86–97.

138. Karbe H, Thiel A, Weber-Luxenburge G et al. Brain plasticity in poststroke aphasia: what is the contribution of the right hemisphere? *Brain Lang* 1998;64(2):215–30.

139. Mimura M, Kato M, Sano Y et al. Prospective and retrospective studies of recovery in aphasia. Changes in cerebral blood flow and language functions. *Brain* 1998;121(Pt 11):2083–94.

140. Mueller RA, Rothermel RD, Behen ME et al. Brain organization of language after early unilateral lesion: a PET study. *Brain Lang* 1998;62(3):422–51.

141. Small SL, Flores DK, Noll DC. Different neural circuits subserve reading before and after therapy for acquired dyslexia. *Brain Lang* 1998;62(2):298–308.

142. Cao Y, Vikingstad EM, George KP et al. Cortical language activation in stroke patients recovering from aphasia with functional MRI. *Stroke* 1999;30:2331–40.

143. Heiss WD, Kessler J, Thiel A et al. Differential capacity of left and right hemispheric areas for compensation of poststroke aphasia. *Ann Neurol* 1999;45:430–8.

144. Miura K, Nakamura Y, Miura F et al. Functional magnetic resonance imaging to word generation task in a patient with Broca´s aphasia. *J Neurol* 1999;246(10):939–42.

145. Musso M, Weiller C, Kiebel S et al. Training-induced brain plasticity in aphasia. *Brain* 1999;122:1781–90.

146. Thulborn KR, Carpenter PA, Just MA. Plasticity of language-related brain function during recovery from stroke. *Stroke* 1999;30:749–54.

147. Warburton E, Price C, Swinburn K et al. Mechanisms of recovery from aphasia: evidence from positron emission tomography studies. *J Neurol Neurosurg Psychiatry* 1999;66:155–61.

148. Calvert GA, Brammer MJ, Morris RG et al. Using fMRI to study recovery from acquired dysphasia. *Brain Lang* 2000;71(3):391–9.

149. Gold BT, Kertesz A. Right hemisphere semantic processing of visual words in an aphasic patient: an fMRI study. *Brain Lang* 2000;73(3):456–65.

150. Binder J. Functional magnetic resonance imaging. Language mapping. *Neurosurg Clin N Am* 1997;8:383–92.

151. Hillis AE, Kane A, Tuffiash E et al. Reperfusion of specific brain regions by raising blood pressure restores selective language functions in subacute stroke. *Brain Lang* 2001;79(3):495–510.

152. Gordon C, Langton-Hewer R, Wade DT. Dysphagia in acute stroke. *BMJ* 1987;295:411–4.

153. Barer DH. The natural history and functional consequences of dysphagia after hemispheric stroke. *J Neurol Neurosurg Psychiatry* 1989;52:236–41.

154. Sumi T. Some properties of cortically-evoked swallowing and chewing in rabbits. *Brain Res* 1969;15(1):107–20.

155. Aziz Q, Rothwell JC, Hamdy S et al. The topographic representation of esophageal motor function on the human cerebral cortex. *Gastroenterology* 1996;111:855–62.

156. Hamdy S, Aziz Q, Rothwell JC et al. The cortical topography of human swallowing musculature in health and disease. *Nat Med* 1996;2(11):1217–24.

157. Hamdy S, Aziz Q, Rothwell JC et al. Explaining oropharyngeal dysphagia after unilateral hemispheric stroke. *Lancet* 1997;350:686–92.

158. Hamdy S, Rothwell JC. Gut feelings about recovery after stroke: the organization and reorganization of human swallowing motor cortex. *Trends Neurosci* 1998;21(7):278–82.

159. Hamdy S, Rothwell JC, Aziz Q et al. Long-term reorganization of human motor cortex driven by short–term sensory stimulation. *Nat Neurosci* 1998;1(1):64–8.

160. Fraser C, Power M, Hamdy S et al. Driving plasticity in human adult motor cortex is associated with improved motor function after brain injury. *Neuron* 2002;34:831–40.

161. Feeney DM, Westerberg VS. Norepinephrine and brain damage: alpha noradrenergic pharmacology alters functional recovery after cortical trauma. *Can J Psychol* 1990;44(2):233–52.

162. Walker-Batson D, Smith P, Curtis S et al. Amphetamine paired with physical therapy accelerates motor recovery after stroke. Further evidence. *Stroke* 1995;26(12):2254–9.

163. Dam M, Tonin P, De Boni A et al. Effects of fluoxetine and maprotiline on functional recovery in poststroke hemiplegic patients undergoing rehabilitation therapy. *Stroke* 1996;27(7):1211–4.

164. Goldstein LB. Pharmacological approach to functional reorganization: the role of norepinephrine. *Rev Neurol (Paris)* 1999;155(9):731–6.

165. Scheidtmann K, Fries W, Muller F et al. Effect of levodopa in combination with physiotherapy on functional motor recovery after stroke: a prospective, randomised, double-blind study. *Lancet* 2001;358(9284):787–90.

9

Abbreviations

2-D	2 dimensional
3-D	3 dimensional
4-D	4 dimensional
DOF	degrees of freedom
ACA	anterior cerebral artery
AD	autosomal dominant
ADC	apparent diffusion coefficient
AHA	American Heart Association
APOE	apolipoprotein E
ASL	arterial spin labeling
ATP	adenosine triphosphate
AV	arteriovenous
AVM	arteriovenous malformation
BA	basilar artery
BDNF	brain-derived neurotropic factor
BZR	benzodiazepine receptor
CAA	cerebral amyloid angiopathy
CBF	cerebral blood flow
CBV	cerebral blood volume
CCA	common carotid artery
CDFI	color Doppler flow imaging
CE	contrast enhanced
CEA	carotid endarterectomy
CHI	contrast harmonic imaging
CIMT	constraint-induced movement therapy
CMR_{glc}	cerebral metabolic rate for glucose
$CMRO_2$	cerebral metabolic rate for oxygen
CSF	cerebrospinal fluid
CT	computed tomography
CTA	computed tomography-angiography

CTP	computed tomography perfusion
CW	continuous wave
DC	direct current
DICE	do not ignore chance effect
DOPA	dihydroxyphenylalanine
DSA	digital subtraction angiography
DTPA	diethylene-triamine penta-acetic acid
DWI	diffusion-weighted imaging
DW-MRI	diffusion-weighted magnetic resonance imaging
ECA	external carotid artery
ECASS II	European Cooperative Acute Stroke Study II
EC-IC	extracranial–intracranial
EEG	electroencephalography
EP	evoked potential(s)
EPI	echoplanar imaging
FDG	fluoro-2-deoxyglucose
FLAIR	fluid-attenuated inversion recovery
fMRI	functional magnetic resonance imaging
FMZ	flumazenil
GABA	gamma-aminobutyric acid
GCS	Glasgow Coma Scale
GEF	glucose extraction fraction
GRE	gradient-recalled echo
HHT	hereditary hemorrhagic telangiectasia
HITS	high-intensity transient signals
HMCAS	hyperdense middle cerebral artery sign
HU	Hounsfield unit
IC	intracerebral cavernous
ICA	internal carotid artery
ICH	intracerebral hemorrhage
ICP	intracranial pressure
IMP	iodoamphetamine
INR	international normalized ratio
LACI	lacunar infarcts
LAD	large artery disease
LSO	lutetium oxyorthosilicate
LSR	Lausanne Stroke Registry
MAL	motor activity log
MCA	middle cerebral artery
MCAO	middle cerebral artery occlusion
MEG	magnetoencephalography

MEP	motor-evoked potential
MES	microembolic signal
MIP	maximal intensity projection
MIT	melodic intonation therapy
MPR	multiplanar reconstruction
MRA	magnetic resonance angiography
MRI	magnetic resonance imaging
MRS	magnetic resonance spectroscopy
MTT	mean transit time
NAA	N-acetyl aspartate
NASCET	North American Symptomatic Carotid Endarterectomy Trial
NIHSS	National Institute of Health Stroke Scale
NINDS	National Institute of Neurological Disorders and Stroke
OCSP	Oxford Community Stroke Project
OEF	oxygen extraction fraction
PACI	partial anterior circulation infarcts
PCA	posterior cerebral artery
PC-MRA	phase contrast MRA
PDI	power Doppler imaging
PET	positron emission tomography
PI	perfusion imaging
PICA	posterior inferior cerebellar artery
PICHI	pulse inversion contrast harmonic imaging
POCI	posterior circulation infarcts
POM	position and orientation measurement
PWI	perfusion-weighted imaging
rCBF	relative cerebral blood flow
rCBV	relative cerebral blood volume
rMTT	relative mean transit time
rTMS	repetitive TMS
rtPA	recombinant tissue plasminogen activator
SAH	subarachnoid hemorrhage
SMA	supplementary motor area
SNR	signal-to-noise ratio
SPECT	single photon emission computed tomography
SWI	susceptibility-weighted imaging
T	tesla (unit of measure of magnetic field strength)
TACI	total anterior circulation infarcts
TCD	transcranial Doppler ultrasonography
TCDFI	transcranial color Doppler flow imaging
TEE	transesophageal echocardiography

TIA	transient ischemic attack
TMS	transcranial magnetic stimulation
TOAST	Trial of ORG 10172 in Acute Stroke Treatment
TOF	time of flight
tPA	tissue plasminogen activator
TTC	tetrazolium chloride
TTP	time to peak
TTT	time to treat
VA	vertebral artery
VSOD	venous sinus occlusive disease

10

Index

A

age, ICH risk factor 128
Albunex, contrast agent 103–104
alcohol, ICH risk factor 128
amputees, cortical reorganization and phantom limb pain 175–176
aneurysm, secondary ICH risk factor 129
anterior cerebral artery (ACA) infarction, CT diagnosis 22–23
anticoagulation therapy
    ICH management 139–140
    ICH risk factor 129
anticonvulsive treatment, ICH 139
antiplatelet therapy, ICH risk factor 129
aphasia
    imaging studies, brain area activations 181–183
    PET studies 161–163
        functional network for recovery 161–163
        left hemispheric speech area activation 161, 162
        left temporal area activation 162–163
        prognosis prediction 160–161
apolipoprotein E gene, ICH risk factor 128, 130, 134
apparent diffusion coefficient (ADC), DWI 48
arteriovenous malformations (AVM)
    contrast-enhanced Doppler sonography 107
    secondary ICH risk factor 129–130
aspirin antiplatelet therapy, ICH risk factor 129
atherosclerosis
    infarction 4, 8
    with stenosis 2
    without stenosis 2, 10